# CARBOHYDRATE
# ADDICT'S
# FAT
# COUNTER

# THE
# CARBOHYDRATE
# ADDICT'S
# FAT
# COUNTER

## DR. RACHAEL F. HELLER
ASSISTANT PROFESSOR EMERITUS, MT. SINAI SCHOOL OF MEDICINE•
ASSISTANT PROFESSOR EMERITUS, GRADUATE CENTER OF THE
CITY UNIVERSITY OF NEW YORK

## DR. RICHARD F. HELLER
PROFESSOR EMERITUS, MT. SINAI SCHOOL OF MEDICINE•
PROFESSOR EMERITUS, GRADUATE CENTER OF THE
CITY UNIVERSITY OF NEW YORK•
PROFESSOR EMERITUS, CITY UNIVERSITY OF NEW YORK

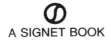

A SIGNET BOOK

A Note to the Reader
The ideas and data contained in this book are not intended as a substitute for medical treatment by a physician. The reader should regularly consult a physician in matters relating to health and prior to any changes in diet.

SIGNET
Published by New American Library, a division of
Penguin Putnam Inc., 375 Hudson Street,
New York, New York 10014, U.S.A.
Penguin Books Ltd, 27 Wrights Lane, London W8 5TZ, England
Penguin Books Australia Ltd, Ringwood, Victoria, Australia
Penguin Books Canada Ltd, 10 Alcorn Avenue, Toronto, Ontario, Canada M4V 3B2
Penguin Books (N.Z.) Ltd, 182–190 Wairau Road, Auckland 10, New Zealand

Penguin Books Ltd, Registered Offices
Harmondsworth, Middlesex, England

First published by Signet, an imprint of New American Library,
a division of Penguin Putnam Inc.

First Printing, January 2000
10  9  8  7  6  5  4

# CONTENTS

In this counter you will find more than 4000 food comparisons* presented in two exciting, easy and reader-friendly formats. The major categories and the page numbers on which you will find them are as follows:

|  | Alphabetical Charts Begin | Hi-Low Comparison Charts Begin |
|---|---|---|

*Nutritional values in this counter were taken from material supplied by or direct communication with the U.S. Department of Agriculture, scientific studies, computer data banks, and representatives of the food industry. When counts, as provided by a variety of sources, differ one from the other, an average or typical count is calculated and used. All data are rounded to the nearest whole number. Neither the authors nor publisher assume any responsibility for any errors contained herein and all readers must work in accordance with and in conjunction with their own personal physician. For information on abbreviations, see the introductory pages that follow.

# INTRODUCTION

**Carbohydrate Indulger or Carbohydrate Addict?**
Carbohydrate addicts have compelling, recurring and intense cravings for starches, snack foods, junk foods, or sweets. Indulgers desire these foods, enjoy them, and walk away. The more often carbohydrate addicts have these foods, the more they crave them—even when they don't want to be eating them. Indulgers choose these foods; carbohydrate addicts sometimes simply lose control. If you are a carbohydrate addict, chances are you respond differently to bread or pasta or potato, to those snack foods or sweets, than do other people. And it's essential that you understand that difference.

Although C. Everett Koop, M.D., the former Surgeon General of the United States, has noted that some of us are "carbohydrate sensitive," some physicians simply don't understand that carbohydrate cravings, weight gain, and health problems can be signs of a powerful hormonal problem. As many as 75 percent of the overweight (and a good percentage of normal-weight individuals as well) appear to have the insulin imbalance that leads to an addiction to carbohydrates. They may never realize that an imbalance in the hormone insulin (known as the "hunger hormone") can make us crave carbohydrate-rich foods intensely and repeatedly.

Yet carbohydrate addiction is not our fault! Our physical makeup, the result of our genetics, make us "too good" at turning carbohydrates into blood fat, then storing it away as body fat, and no matter how great our willpower, our bodies seem to fight us at every level. An imbalance of insulin can make carbohydrate-rich foods taste exceptionally good and can increase our ability and tendency to put on weight and to keep it on as well. We now understand what causes carbohydrate addiction and are happy to say that we know how to correct it as well.

It is essential to understand that carbohydrate addiction is not a matter of willpower but rather a matter of biology; a carbohydrate addict's cravings and weight gain are little more than symptoms of an underlying physical imbalance—a simple case of having the right body in the wrong time; a caveman's body in a modern world of plenty.

## Are you addicted to carbohydrates?

yes  no  Do you have a difficult time stopping, once you start to eat starches, snack foods, junk foods, or sweets?

yes  no  After a full breakfast, do you get hungrier before it's time for lunch?

yes  no  Do you get tired and/or hungry in the mid-afternoon and find that a snack makes you feel better?

yes  no  Do you put weight on easily or, after dieting, tend to gain weight back quickly?

yes  no  Do you continue to eat or snack even when you are not really hungry?

yes  no  Do you sometimes lose control of your eating?

Two or more yes answers? You may very well be carbohydrate addicted!

If you are addicted to carbohydrates, we can explain why you have struggled to stay on diet after diet, why diets often fail to help you keep the weight off, and why your health and happiness may have suffered. For the carbohydrate addict, starches, snack foods, junk foods and sweets may hold the key to your addiction and to your victory as well. On our Programs, you will find that you can enjoy the foods you love and need every day.

For our Programs' essential guidelines, see *The Carbohydrate Addict's LifeSpan Program* (Plume), *The Carbohydrate Addict's*

*Healthy for Life Plan* (Plume), *The Carbohydrate Addict's Diet* (Signet) or *The Carbohydrate Addict's Healthy Heart Program* (Ballantine). Our companion workbook, *The Carbohydrate Addict's Program for Success* (Plume), offers help with the emotional and spiritual aspects of carbohydrate addiction and our other *Carbohydrate Addict's Counters* (Signet) of graphically formatted information charts can provide vital facts for success.

## A Message from Drs. Richard and Rachael Heller

We have both fought "the battle of the bulge" for as long as we can remember. We spent our childhoods learning the caloric content of foods and struggling to master the calorie counters of the time.

The calorie counters of our childhood, however, were barely usable. Never-ending columns and rows of tiny numbers filled page after page, offering few insights and little real help.

As overweight adults, when we attempted to control our intake of dietary fat, we found ourselves confronted with the same boring and unrewarding rows of numbers. We would face the almost herculean task of making informed choices when the data simply did not allow for intelligent comparisons. The fat content of one soup might be listed on the same page as the fat content of twenty other soups but, much to our confusion, several of the soups differed widely in portion (one cup versus one can; milk added versus water). No comparisons were possible without involved calculations. Many authors of gram counters have found it easy and fast to use noncomparable portions published in already-available databases. At the time, we as authors simply felt confused and frustrated.

Like so many people, we blamed ourselves rather than authors of the gram counters that failed to provide us with the usable information we needed to succeed.

Today we have been given an opportunity to make things better! In the books that make up our Carbohydrate Addict's Counters series, you will find that the calorie, carbohydrate, and fat content of foods, respectively, are simple to see and easy to compare.

With these new, revolutionary gram counters, you will be able to walk into a fast food restaurant or down your favorite supermarket aisle and feel like you are in control—because you will be. You will be able to make calorie-, carbohydrate-, and fat-related choices in an instant and feel free of nagging doubts and guilt.

And, most importantly, with each success you achieve, you will grow more confident.

No thanks to old gram counters, we have now lost a combined weight of more than two hundred pounds and we have maintained our ideal weight and health for over fifteen years. We are happier than we ever thought we could be and we are healthier and more energetic as well.

Our hope is that, in writing this new series of gram counters, you too will discover the joy that comes as the challenges and frustration of the past are replaced by successes of the present (and future). The struggles of the past make today's victories even sweeter.

    With our warmest wishes,
    Drs. Richard and Rachael Heller

## Two Roads, One Goal: Success

In the pages that follow you will discover two unique, fun, and easy formats to help you in your gram counting—two types of charts that will help put you in charge of making your fat-related food choices.

Alphabetical Charts make up the first half of this book. These charts will allow you to locate a specific food item by its name from A to Z, within its food group. Alphabetical Charts will make it easy for you to see, at a glance, how high your food choice is with regard to fat content and how it compares to other foods within that same group. Alphabetical Charts will help you to decide if the fat content of your food makes it a good selection for you. While the bars on each Alphabetical Chart illustrate the amount of fat content of each food, the number at the end of each bar will provide you with the specific level of fat content.

You will find Hi-Low Comparison Charts in the second half of the book. Hi-Low Comparison Charts will help you compare foods within a given group and visualize the fat content of a given food group—from high to low and all those in between.

Hi-Low Comparison Charts can provide you with suggestions on what to eat while keeping your dietary fat levels low.

## What Is a Dietary Fat?

Fat is one of the body's necessary nutrients (the others being carbohydrates and proteins). All forms of fat are made up of a combination of building blocks called fatty acids. These building blocks can remain unattached as single molecules (free fatty acids) or may be assembled into groupings that form larger molecules (fats). A saturated fat is a fat in which each molecule in the group of molecules that makes up a fat is filled to capacity with hydrogen. When there is one opening for an atom in each molecule, the fat is said to be monounsaturated. When there are several openings for hydrogen in each molecule, the fat is said to be polyunsaturated.

A handy guideline you can use is that saturated fats generally come from animal sources and usually remain solid at room temperature. Some tropical oils, such as coconut oil and palm oil, are exceptions to the solid-saturated-fat rule. These two saturated oils are semi-solid at room temperature and come from plant sources.

A diet high in saturated fats has been shown to increase the risk of heart disease and some forms of cancer. It is important to remember that it is not advisable to make any changes in your dietary choices without first discussing the matter with your physician.

## How Much Fat Should I Eat?

The American Heart Association in their Eating Plan for Healthy Americans offers the following nutritional guidelines:

- **Total fat** intake should be no more than 30 percent of total calories.
- **Saturated fatty acid** intake should be 8–10 percent of total calories.
- **Polyunsaturated fatty acid** intake should be up to 10 percent of total calories.
- **Monounsaturated fatty acids** make up to 15 percent of total calories.
- **Cholesterol** intake should be less than 300 milligrams per day.

As always, individual needs must be considered, so check with your physician before making any dietary or lifestyle changes.

For purposes of calculation, each gram of fat contains 9 calories.

## Am I Overweight?

While there is no definitive way to determine whether you are at your ideal weight, here are three weight check-ups to help you decide.

## Check-up #1: Are You in the Range?

The chart that follows is a standardized chart used by the United States Department of Agriculture.

## Check-up #2: Can You Pinch an Inch?

While weight range charts can help you to settle the weight-loss question, standardized charts can fail to take many variables into account. A simple and quick test for determining excess body fat is to pinch a fold of skin at the back of your upper arm. If you can pinch more than an inch, you are probably carrying more weight (in the form of fat) than is desirable.

## Check-up #3: What's Your Body Mass Index (BMI)?

Body Mass Index Scores can prove a good indicator of an individual's weight level. The BMI uses a mathematical formula

## RANGE OF "DESIRABLE" WEIGHTS*

| Height without shoes | Weight without clothes | |
| --- | --- | --- |
| | Men (pounds) | Women (pounds) |
| 4'10" | | 92–121 |
| 4'11" | | 95–124 |
| 5'0" | | 98–127 |
| 5'1" | 105–134 | 101–130 |
| 5'2" | 108–137 | 104–134 |
| 5'3" | 111–141 | 107–138 |
| 5'4" | 114–145 | 110–142 |
| 5'5" | 117–149 | 114–146 |
| 5'6" | 121–154 | 118–150 |
| 5'7" | 125–159 | 122–154 |
| 5'8" | 129–163 | 126–159 |
| 5'9" | 133–167 | 130–164 |
| 5'10" | 137–172 | 134–169 |
| 5'11" | 141–177 | |
| 6'0" | 145–182 | |
| 6'1" | 149–187 | |
| 6'2" | 153–192 | |
| 6'3" | 157–197 | |

*United States Department of Agriculture Human Nutrition Information Service Agriculture, Information Bulletin 364.

that takes into account both a person's weight and height. BMI equals a person's weight in kilograms divided by height in meters squared (BMI=kg/m$^2$). No need to run for the calculator though. On the following page is a table that will make it easy for you to get your BMI score.

To use the BMI table, find your height in the left-hand column. Move across the row to your weight. The number at the bottom of the column is your Body Mass Index (BMI).

# BODY MASS INDEX (BMI) CHART

Height (in.)

| Height (in.) | | | | | | | | | | | | | | |
|---|---|---|---|---|---|---|---|---|---|---|---|---|---|---|
| 58 | 91 | 96 | 100 | 105 | 110 | 115 | 119 | 124 | 129 | 134 | 138 | 143 | 167 | 191 |
| 59 | 94 | 99 | 104 | 109 | 114 | 119 | 124 | 128 | 133 | 138 | 143 | 148 | 173 | 198 |
| 60 | 97 | 102 | 107 | 112 | 118 | 123 | 128 | 133 | 138 | 143 | 148 | 153 | 179 | 204 |
| 61 | 100 | 106 | 111 | 116 | 122 | 127 | 132 | 137 | 143 | 148 | 153 | 158 | 185 | 211 |
| 62 | 104 | 109 | 115 | 120 | 126 | 131 | 136 | 142 | 147 | 153 | 158 | 164 | 191 | 218 |
| 63 | 107 | 113 | 118 | 124 | 130 | 135 | 141 | 146 | 152 | 158 | 163 | 169 | 197 | 225 |
| 64 | 110 | 116 | 122 | 128 | 134 | 140 | 145 | 151 | 157 | 163 | 169 | 174 | 204 | 232 |
| 65 | 114 | 120 | 126 | 132 | 138 | 144 | 150 | 156 | 162 | 168 | 174 | 180 | 210 | 240 |
| 66 | 118 | 124 | 130 | 136 | 142 | 148 | 155 | 161 | 167 | 173 | 179 | 186 | 216 | 247 |
| 67 | 121 | 127 | 134 | 140 | 146 | 153 | 159 | 166 | 172 | 178 | 185 | 191 | 223 | 255 |
| 68 | 125 | 131 | 138 | 144 | 151 | 158 | 164 | 171 | 177 | 184 | 190 | 197 | 230 | 262 |
| 69 | 128 | 135 | 142 | 149 | 155 | 162 | 169 | 176 | 182 | 189 | 196 | 203 | 236 | 270 |
| 70 | 132 | 139 | 146 | 153 | 160 | 167 | 174 | 181 | 188 | 195 | 202 | 207 | 243 | 278 |
| 71 | 136 | 143 | 150 | 157 | 165 | 172 | 179 | 186 | 193 | 200 | 208 | 215 | 250 | 286 |
| 72 | 140 | 147 | 154 | 162 | 169 | 177 | 184 | 191 | 199 | 206 | 213 | 221 | 258 | 294 |
| 73 | 144 | 151 | 159 | 166 | 174 | 182 | 189 | 197 | 204 | 212 | 219 | 227 | 265 | 302 |
| 74 | 148 | 155 | 163 | 171 | 179 | 186 | 194 | 202 | 210 | 218 | 225 | 233 | 272 | 311 |
| 75 | 152 | 160 | 168 | 176 | 184 | 192 | 200 | 208 | 216 | 224 | 232 | 240 | 279 | 319 |
| 76 | 156 | 164 | 172 | 180 | 189 | 197 | 205 | 213 | 221 | 230 | 238 | 246 | 287 | 328 |
| BMI (kg/m$^2$) | 19 | 20 | 21 | 22 | 23 | 24 | 25 | 26 | 27 | 28 | 29 | 30 | 35 | 40 |

Using your BMI score, the chart below can help you to better determine your weight level.

| BMI (Body Mass Index) | Weight Assessment |
|---|---|
| 18.5 or less | Underweight |
| 18.5–24.9 | Normal |
| 25.0–29.9 | Overweight |
| 30.0–39.9 | Obese |
| 40 or greater | Extremely Obese |

## TO OUR READERS: AN IMPORTANT NOTE

We hope that this counter will become a good and well-used friend. It carries with it the experiences of over half a million people along with our best wishes for a long, healthy, and happy life.

Any change in diet should be made in consultation with your physician. The data contained herein are not intended to replace medical advice. Any questions or concerns should be addressed to your physician.

## IN YOUR HANDS

In your hands you hold the information you will need to make intelligent and informed choices—important decisions that can make your health and weight-related dreams come true. But, beyond this book, you hold within your hands the future that is yet to be.

You can shape that future by staying focused on your goals and by listening to your heart, mind, and body. They have much to tell us . . . when we listen.

The best thing about the future is just that. It lies ahead, beckoning us to follow and explore. In that adventure we call life, we wish you the best . . . from the world around and the world within as well.

## ABBREVIATIONS YOU'LL FIND IN
## THE CARBOHYDRATE ADDICT'S COUNTERS

| When You See This Abbreviation. . . . | It Means This |
|---|---|
| / | or |
| w/ | with |
| bl cheese | blue cheese |
| broc | broccoli |
| ch | cheese |
| dress | dressing |
| env | envelope |
| fl | fluid or flavor |
| flav | flavor(s) |
| Fr dress | French dressing |
| frzn | frozen |
| G'ma's Big | Grandma's Big |
| marg | margarine |
| parm | parmesan |
| Pepperidge | Pepperidge Farm |
| pkg | package |
| pkt | packet |
| q'tr pnd'r | quarter pounder |
| reg | regular |
| saus | sausage |
| Stella D | Stella D'Oro |
| sweet'd | sweetened |
| Thous Island | Thousand Island |
| tom | tomato |
| veg | vegetable |
| wh | white |

# THE
# CARBOHYDRATE
# ADDICT'S
# FAT
# COUNTER

# ALPHABETICAL CHARTS

## BEVERAGES*, Part 1

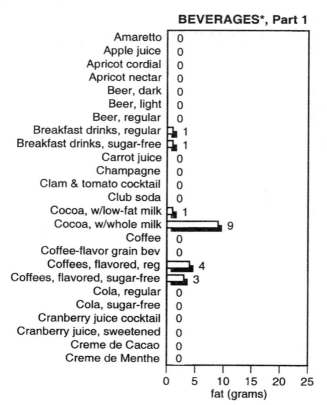

| | fat (grams) |
|---|---|
| Amaretto | 0 |
| Apple juice | 0 |
| Apricot cordial | 0 |
| Apricot nectar | 0 |
| Beer, dark | 0 |
| Beer, light | 0 |
| Beer, regular | 0 |
| Breakfast drinks, regular | 1 |
| Breakfast drinks, sugar-free | 1 |
| Carrot juice | 0 |
| Champagne | 0 |
| Clam & tomato cocktail | 0 |
| Club soda | 0 |
| Cocoa, w/low-fat milk | 1 |
| Cocoa, w/whole milk | 9 |
| Coffee | 0 |
| Coffee-flavor grain bev | 0 |
| Coffees, flavored, reg | 4 |
| Coffees, flavored, sugar-free | 3 |
| Cola, regular | 0 |
| Cola, sugar-free | 0 |
| Cranberry juice cocktail | 0 |
| Cranberry juice, sweetened | 0 |
| Creme de Cacao | 0 |
| Creme de Menthe | 0 |

0   5   10   15   20   25
fat (grams)

\* Counts for non-alcoholic drinks and beer are based on
8-fluid-ounce servings, for wine on 3 1/2-fluid-ounce
servings and, for hard liquor, on 1 1/2-fluid-ounce servings.

2

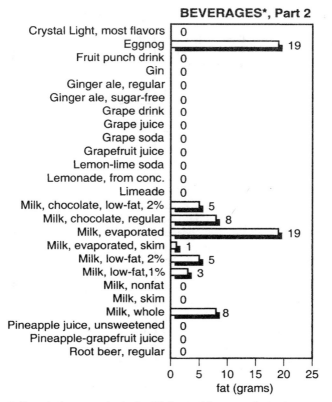

**BEVERAGES\*, Part 2**

| | fat (grams) |
|---|---|
| Crystal Light, most flavors | 0 |
| Eggnog | 19 |
| Fruit punch drink | 0 |
| Gin | 0 |
| Ginger ale, regular | 0 |
| Ginger ale, sugar-free | 0 |
| Grape drink | 0 |
| Grape juice | 0 |
| Grape soda | 0 |
| Grapefruit juice | 0 |
| Lemon-lime soda | 0 |
| Lemonade, from conc. | 0 |
| Limeade | 0 |
| Milk, chocolate, low-fat, 2% | 5 |
| Milk, chocolate, regular | 8 |
| Milk, evaporated | 19 |
| Milk, evaporated, skim | 1 |
| Milk, low-fat, 2% | 5 |
| Milk, low-fat,1% | 3 |
| Milk, nonfat | 0 |
| Milk, skim | 0 |
| Milk, whole | 8 |
| Pineapple juice, unsweetened | 0 |
| Pineapple-grapefruit juice | 0 |
| Root beer, regular | 0 |

0    5    10    15    20    25
fat (grams)

\* Counts for non-alcoholic drinks and beer are based on
8-fluid-ounce servings, for wine on 3 1/2-fluid-ounce
servings and, for hard liquor, on 1 1/2-fluid-ounce servings.

3

## BEVERAGES*, Part 3

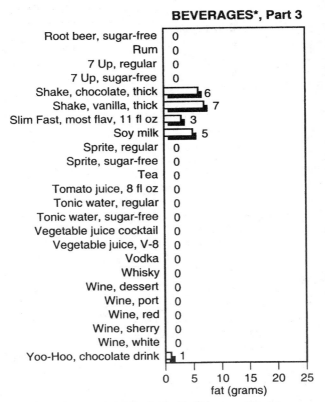

| | fat (grams) |
|---|---|
| Root beer, sugar-free | 0 |
| Rum | 0 |
| 7 Up, regular | 0 |
| 7 Up, sugar-free | 0 |
| Shake, chocolate, thick | 6 |
| Shake, vanilla, thick | 7 |
| Slim Fast, most flav, 11 fl oz | 3 |
| Soy milk | 5 |
| Sprite, regular | 0 |
| Sprite, sugar-free | 0 |
| Tea | 0 |
| Tomato juice, 8 fl oz | 0 |
| Tonic water, regular | 0 |
| Tonic water, sugar-free | 0 |
| Vegetable juice cocktail | 0 |
| Vegetable juice, V-8 | 0 |
| Vodka | 0 |
| Whisky | 0 |
| Wine, dessert | 0 |
| Wine, port | 0 |
| Wine, red | 0 |
| Wine, sherry | 0 |
| Wine, white | 0 |
| Yoo-Hoo, chocolate drink | 1 |

0   5   10   15   20   25
fat (grams)

* Counts for non-alcoholic drinks and beer are based on
8-fluid-ounce servings, for wine on 3 1/2-fluid-ounce
servings and, for hard liquor, on 1 1/2-fluid-ounce servings.

4

## Bread, Crackers, and Flours:
## BAGELS*

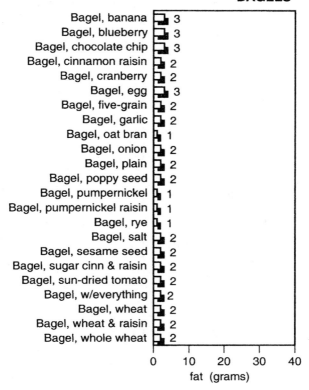

| | |
|---|---|
| Bagel, banana | 3 |
| Bagel, blueberry | 3 |
| Bagel, chocolate chip | 3 |
| Bagel, cinnamon raisin | 2 |
| Bagel, cranberry | 2 |
| Bagel, egg | 3 |
| Bagel, five-grain | 2 |
| Bagel, garlic | 2 |
| Bagel, oat bran | 1 |
| Bagel, onion | 2 |
| Bagel, plain | 2 |
| Bagel, poppy seed | 2 |
| Bagel, pumpernickel | 1 |
| Bagel, pumpernickel raisin | 1 |
| Bagel, rye | 1 |
| Bagel, salt | 2 |
| Bagel, sesame seed | 2 |
| Bagel, sugar cinn & raisin | 2 |
| Bagel, sun-dried tomato | 2 |
| Bagel, w/everything | 2 |
| Bagel, wheat | 2 |
| Bagel, wheat & raisin | 2 |
| Bagel, whole wheat | 2 |

fat (grams)

\* Counts are based on one bagel, approximate weight:
3 ounces.

### Bread, Crackers, and Flours:
### BISCUITS, ROLLS & MUFFINS*

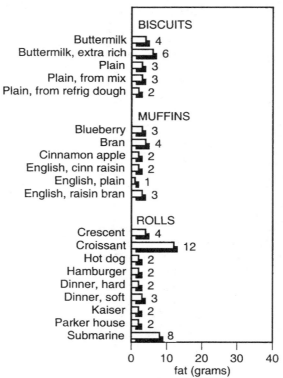

BISCUITS

| | |
|---|---|
| Buttermilk | 4 |
| Buttermilk, extra rich | 6 |
| Plain | 3 |
| Plain, from mix | 3 |
| Plain, from refrig dough | 2 |

MUFFINS

| | |
|---|---|
| Blueberry | 3 |
| Bran | 4 |
| Cinnamon apple | 2 |
| English, cinn raisin | 2 |
| English, plain | 1 |
| English, raisin bran | 3 |

ROLLS

| | |
|---|---|
| Crescent | 4 |
| Croissant | 12 |
| Hot dog | 2 |
| Hamburger | 2 |
| Dinner, hard | 2 |
| Dinner, soft | 3 |
| Kaiser | 2 |
| Parker house | 2 |
| Submarine | 8 |

0    10    20    30    40
fat (grams)

\* Counts are based on single, average-size items. Average
sweet muffin is assumed to be 2 3/4 inches by 2 inches.
Average sweet and English muffin weight is 57 grams.

6

## Bread, Crackers, and Flours:
## BREAD*

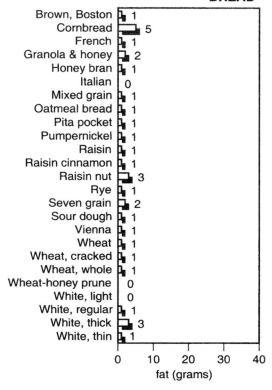

| Bread | fat (grams) |
|---|---|
| Brown, Boston | 1 |
| Cornbread | 5 |
| French | 1 |
| Granola & honey | 2 |
| Honey bran | 1 |
| Italian | 0 |
| Mixed grain | 1 |
| Oatmeal bread | 1 |
| Pita pocket | 1 |
| Pumpernickel | 1 |
| Raisin | 1 |
| Raisin cinnamon | 1 |
| Raisin nut | 3 |
| Rye | 1 |
| Seven grain | 2 |
| Sour dough | 1 |
| Vienna | 1 |
| Wheat | 1 |
| Wheat, cracked | 1 |
| Wheat, whole | 1 |
| Wheat-honey prune | 0 |
| White, light | 0 |
| White, regular | 1 |
| White, thick | 3 |
| White, thin | 1 |

fat (grams)

\* Counts are based on single, average-size slices.

7

## Bread, Crackers, and Flours:
## CRACKERS*

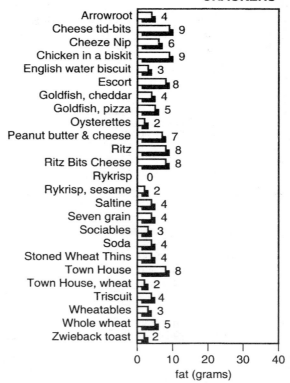

| Cracker | fat (grams) |
|---|---|
| Arrowroot | 4 |
| Cheese tid-bits | 9 |
| Cheeze Nip | 6 |
| Chicken in a biskit | 9 |
| English water biscuit | 3 |
| Escort | 8 |
| Goldfish, cheddar | 4 |
| Goldfish, pizza | 5 |
| Oysterettes | 2 |
| Peanut butter & cheese | 7 |
| Ritz | 8 |
| Ritz Bits Cheese | 8 |
| Rykrisp | 0 |
| Rykrisp, sesame | 2 |
| Saltine | 4 |
| Seven grain | 4 |
| Sociables | 3 |
| Soda | 4 |
| Stoned Wheat Thins | 4 |
| Town House | 8 |
| Town House, wheat | 2 |
| Triscuit | 4 |
| Wheatables | 3 |
| Whole wheat | 5 |
| Zwieback toast | 2 |

fat (grams) — 0 10 20 30 40

\* For ease of comparison, counts are based on one-ounce servings. Adjust counts to reflect quantities consumed.

## Bread, Crackers, and Flours:
## DRY & CRISPY*

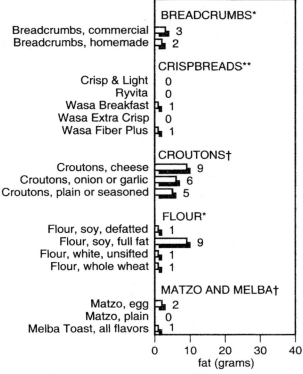

BREADCRUMBS*

Breadcrumbs, commercial 3
Breadcrumbs, homemade 2

CRISPBREADS**

Crisp & Light 0
Ryvita 0
Wasa Breakfast 1
Wasa Extra Crisp 0
Wasa Fiber Plus 1

CROUTONS†

Croutons, cheese 9
Croutons, onion or garlic 6
Croutons, plain or seasoned 5

FLOUR*

Flour, soy, defatted 1
Flour, soy, full fat 9
Flour, white, unsifted 1
Flour, whole wheat 1

MATZO AND MELBA†

Matzo, egg 2
Matzo, plain 0
Melba Toast, all flavors 1

0    10    20    30    40
fat (grams)

* Counts are based on 1/2- cup servings.
** Counts are based on single item.
† Counts are based on single-ounce servings.

## Bread, Crackers, and Flours:
## PANCAKES, STUFFING & MORE*

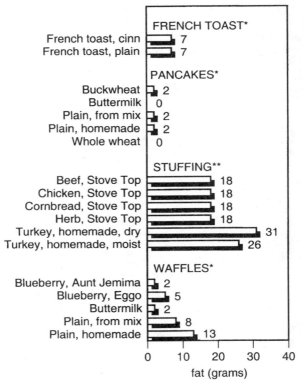

**FRENCH TOAST***

| | |
|---|---|
| French toast, cinn | 7 |
| French toast, plain | 7 |

**PANCAKES***

| | |
|---|---|
| Buckwheat | 2 |
| Buttermilk | 0 |
| Plain, from mix | 2 |
| Plain, homemade | 2 |
| Whole wheat | 0 |

**STUFFING****

| | |
|---|---|
| Beef, Stove Top | 18 |
| Chicken, Stove Top | 18 |
| Cornbread, Stove Top | 18 |
| Herb, Stove Top | 18 |
| Turkey, homemade, dry | 31 |
| Turkey, homemade, moist | 26 |

**WAFFLES***

| | |
|---|---|
| Blueberry, Aunt Jemima | 2 |
| Blueberry, Eggo | 5 |
| Buttermilk | 2 |
| Plain, from mix | 8 |
| Plain, homemade | 13 |

0   10   20   30   40

fat (grams)

\* Counts are based on single slice, pancake, or waffle.
\*\* Counts are based on 1/2-cup servings, prepared.

**CEREALS\*, Part 1**

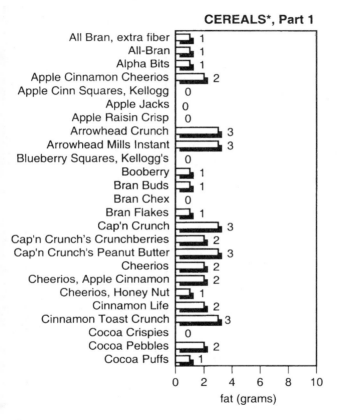

| Cereal | fat (grams) |
|---|---|
| All Bran, extra fiber | 1 |
| All-Bran | 1 |
| Alpha Bits | 1 |
| Apple Cinnamon Cheerios | 2 |
| Apple Cinn Squares, Kellogg | 0 |
| Apple Jacks | 0 |
| Apple Raisin Crisp | 0 |
| Arrowhead Crunch | 3 |
| Arrowhead Mills Instant | 3 |
| Blueberry Squares, Kellogg's | 0 |
| Booberry | 1 |
| Bran Buds | 1 |
| Bran Chex | 0 |
| Bran Flakes | 1 |
| Cap'n Crunch | 3 |
| Cap'n Crunch's Crunchberries | 2 |
| Cap'n Crunch's Peanut Butter | 3 |
| Cheerios | 2 |
| Cheerios, Apple Cinnamon | 2 |
| Cheerios, Honey Nut | 1 |
| Cinnamon Life | 2 |
| Cinnamon Toast Crunch | 3 |
| Cocoa Crispies | 0 |
| Cocoa Pebbles | 2 |
| Cocoa Puffs | 1 |

fat (grams)

\* Counts are based on average-size servings (as indicated
on package) and without added milk.

11

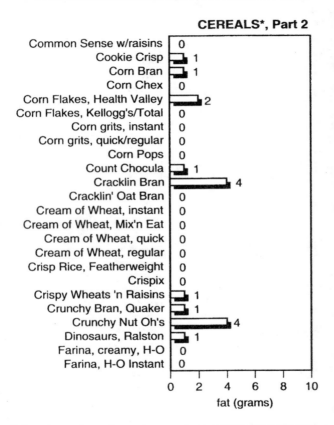

## CEREALS*, Part 2

| | fat (grams) |
|---|---|
| Common Sense w/raisins | 0 |
| Cookie Crisp | 1 |
| Corn Bran | 1 |
| Corn Chex | 0 |
| Corn Flakes, Health Valley | 2 |
| Corn Flakes, Kellogg's/Total | 0 |
| Corn grits, instant | 0 |
| Corn grits, quick/regular | 0 |
| Corn Pops | 0 |
| Count Chocula | 1 |
| Cracklin Bran | 4 |
| Cracklin' Oat Bran | 0 |
| Cream of Wheat, instant | 0 |
| Cream of Wheat, Mix'n Eat | 0 |
| Cream of Wheat, quick | 0 |
| Cream of Wheat, regular | 0 |
| Crisp Rice, Featherweight | 0 |
| Crispix | 0 |
| Crispy Wheats 'n Raisins | 1 |
| Crunchy Bran, Quaker | 1 |
| Crunchy Nut Oh's | 4 |
| Dinosaurs, Ralston | 1 |
| Farina, creamy, H-O | 0 |
| Farina, H-O Instant | 0 |

* Counts are based on average-size servings (as indicated
on package) and without added milk.

12

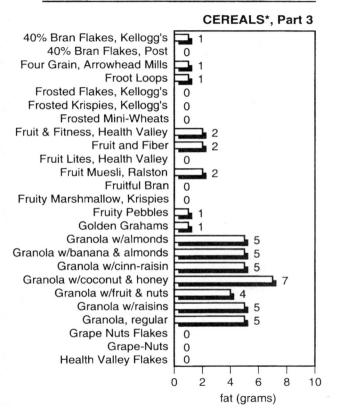

## Alphabetical Chart
(for Hi-Low Comparison Charts, see pages 83 - 164)

### CEREALS*, Part 3

| Cereal | fat (grams) |
|---|---|
| 40% Bran Flakes, Kellogg's | 1 |
| 40% Bran Flakes, Post | 0 |
| Four Grain, Arrowhead Mills | 1 |
| Froot Loops | 1 |
| Frosted Flakes, Kellogg's | 0 |
| Frosted Krispies, Kellogg's | 0 |
| Frosted Mini-Wheats | 0 |
| Fruit & Fitness, Health Valley | 2 |
| Fruit and Fiber | 2 |
| Fruit Lites, Health Valley | 0 |
| Fruit Muesli, Ralston | 2 |
| Fruitful Bran | 0 |
| Fruity Marshmallow, Krispies | 0 |
| Fruity Pebbles | 1 |
| Golden Grahams | 1 |
| Granola w/almonds | 5 |
| Granola w/banana & almonds | 5 |
| Granola w/cinn-raisin | 5 |
| Granola w/coconut & honey | 7 |
| Granola w/fruit & nuts | 4 |
| Granola w/raisins | 5 |
| Granola, regular | 5 |
| Grape Nuts Flakes | 0 |
| Grape-Nuts | 0 |
| Health Valley Flakes | 0 |

fat (grams)

* Counts are based on average-size servings (as indicated
on package) and without added milk.

13

## CEREALS*, Part 4

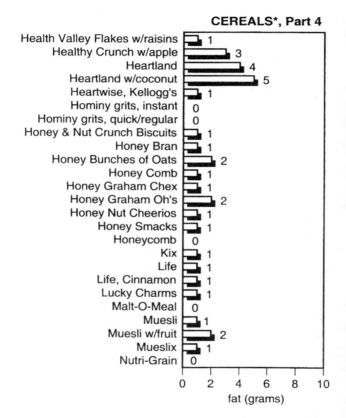

| Cereal | fat (grams) |
|---|---|
| Health Valley Flakes w/raisins | 1 |
| Healthy Crunch w/apple | 3 |
| Heartland | 4 |
| Heartland w/coconut | 5 |
| Heartwise, Kellogg's | 1 |
| Hominy grits, instant | 0 |
| Hominy grits, quick/regular | 0 |
| Honey & Nut Crunch Biscuits | 1 |
| Honey Bran | 1 |
| Honey Bunches of Oats | 2 |
| Honey Comb | 1 |
| Honey Graham Chex | 1 |
| Honey Graham Oh's | 2 |
| Honey Nut Cheerios | 1 |
| Honey Smacks | 1 |
| Honeycomb | 0 |
| Kix | 1 |
| Life | 1 |
| Life, Cinnamon | 1 |
| Lucky Charms | 1 |
| Malt-O-Meal | 0 |
| Muesli | 1 |
| Muesli w/fruit | 2 |
| Mueslix | 1 |
| Nutri-Grain | 0 |

* Counts are based on average-size servings (as indicated
on package) and without added milk.

## CEREALS*, Part 5

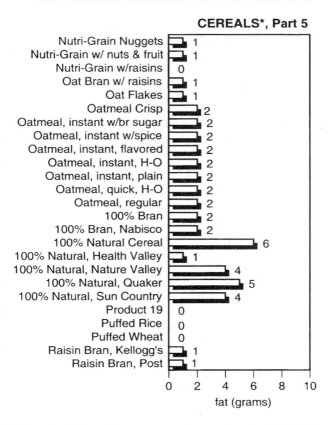

| Cereal | fat (grams) |
|---|---|
| Nutri-Grain Nuggets | 1 |
| Nutri-Grain w/ nuts & fruit | 1 |
| Nutri-Grain w/raisins | 0 |
| Oat Bran w/ raisins | 1 |
| Oat Flakes | 1 |
| Oatmeal Crisp | 2 |
| Oatmeal, instant w/br sugar | 2 |
| Oatmeal, instant w/spice | 2 |
| Oatmeal, instant, flavored | 2 |
| Oatmeal, instant, H-O | 2 |
| Oatmeal, instant, plain | 2 |
| Oatmeal, quick, H-O | 2 |
| Oatmeal, regular | 2 |
| 100% Bran | 2 |
| 100% Bran, Nabisco | 2 |
| 100% Natural Cereal | 6 |
| 100% Natural, Health Valley | 1 |
| 100% Natural, Nature Valley | 4 |
| 100% Natural, Quaker | 5 |
| 100% Natural, Sun Country | 4 |
| Product 19 | 0 |
| Puffed Rice | 0 |
| Puffed Wheat | 0 |
| Raisin Bran, Kellogg's | 1 |
| Raisin Bran, Post | 1 |

fat (grams)

* Counts are based on average-size servings (as indicated
on package) and without added milk.

15

**CEREALS, Part 6**

| Cereal | fat (grams) |
|---|---|
| Raisin Bran, Total | 1 |
| Raisin Nut Bran | 3 |
| Raisin Oat Bran, General Mills | 1 |
| Raisin Squares, Kellogg's | 0 |
| Rice Bran, Health Valley | 1 |
| Rice Chex | 0 |
| Rice Krispies | 0 |
| Seven Grain, Arrowhead Mills | 1 |
| Shredded Wheat, Nabisco | 1 |
| Shredded Wheat, Nutri-Grain | 0 |
| Shredded Wheat, Quaker | 0 |
| Smurf-Magic Berries | 1 |
| Special K | 0 |
| Sugar Smacks | 1 |
| Super Golden Crisps | 0 |
| Super Sugar Crisp | 0 |
| Toasties, Post | 0 |
| Total | 1 |
| Total Quick | 2 |
| Trix | 0 |
| Wheat Chex | 0 |
| Wheat Flakes | 1 |
| Wheatena | 1 |
| Wheaties | 0 |

fat (grams): 0  2  4  6  8  10

\* Counts are based on average-size servings (as indicated on package) and without added milk.

## COMBINED AND FROZEN FOODS*,
## Part 1

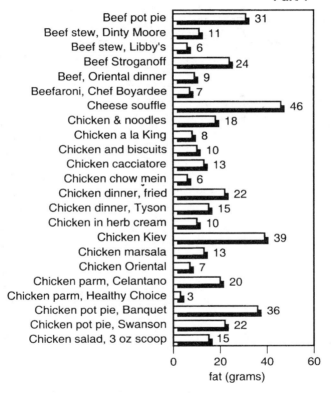

| Food | fat (grams) |
|------|-------------|
| Beef pot pie | 31 |
| Beef stew, Dinty Moore | 11 |
| Beef stew, Libby's | 6 |
| Beef Stroganoff | 24 |
| Beef, Oriental dinner | 9 |
| Beefaroni, Chef Boyardee | 7 |
| Cheese souffle | 46 |
| Chicken & noodles | 18 |
| Chicken a la King | 8 |
| Chicken and biscuits | 10 |
| Chicken cacciatore | 13 |
| Chicken chow mein | 6 |
| Chicken dinner, fried | 22 |
| Chicken dinner, Tyson | 15 |
| Chicken in herb cream | 10 |
| Chicken Kiev | 39 |
| Chicken marsala | 13 |
| Chicken Oriental | 7 |
| Chicken parm, Celantano | 20 |
| Chicken parm, Healthy Choice | 3 |
| Chicken pot pie, Banquet | 36 |
| Chicken pot pie, Swanson | 22 |
| Chicken salad, 3 oz scoop | 15 |

fat (grams) — 0    20    40    60

\* Counts are based on average-size servings as indicated
on package. Adjust count to reflect amount consumed.

## COMBINED AND FROZEN FOODS*,
### Part 2

| Food | fat (grams) |
|------|-------------|
| Chili, w/beans, Hormel | 17 |
| Chili, w/beans, most brands | 16 |
| Chili, no beans, Dennison's | 20 |
| Chili, no beans, Hormel | 32 |
| Chop suey | 17 |
| Chopped sirloin | 16 |
| Cinnamon swirls w/sausage | 21 |
| Corned beef hash, canned | 26 |
| Crabs, devilled, 2 | 16 |
| Dinosaurs, Chef Boyardee | 10 |
| Egg roll, chicken | 8 |
| Egg roll, pork | 6 |
| Egg roll, vegetarian | 6 |
| Enchilada, beef | 15 |
| Enchilada, cheese | 19 |
| Enchilada, chicken | 18 |
| Fajita, beef | 14 |
| Fettuccini Alfredo | 13 |
| Fettuccini w/meat sauce | 12 |
| Fish & chips | 25 |
| Fried rice w/chicken/pork | 4 |
| Green pepper stuffed w/beef | 9 |
| Ham and cheese pocket, frzn | 16 |

0   20   40   60
fat (grams)

* Counts are based on average-size servings as indicated
on package. Adjust count to reflect amount consumed.

18

## COMBINED AND FROZEN FOODS*,
## Part 3

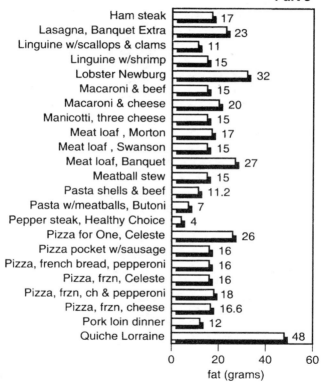

| Food | fat (grams) |
|------|-------------|
| Ham steak | 17 |
| Lasagna, Banquet Extra | 23 |
| Linguine w/scallops & clams | 11 |
| Linguine w/shrimp | 15 |
| Lobster Newburg | 32 |
| Macaroni & beef | 15 |
| Macaroni & cheese | 20 |
| Manicotti, three cheese | 15 |
| Meat loaf , Morton | 17 |
| Meat loaf , Swanson | 15 |
| Meat loaf, Banquet | 27 |
| Meatball stew | 15 |
| Pasta shells & beef | 11.2 |
| Pasta w/meatballs, Butoni | 7 |
| Pepper steak, Healthy Choice | 4 |
| Pizza for One, Celeste | 26 |
| Pizza pocket w/sausage | 16 |
| Pizza, french bread, pepperoni | 16 |
| Pizza, frzn, Celeste | 16 |
| Pizza, frzn, ch & pepperoni | 18 |
| Pizza, frzn, cheese | 16.6 |
| Pork loin dinner | 12 |
| Quiche Lorraine | 48 |

* Counts are based on average-size servings as indicated
on package. Adjust count to reflect amount consumed.

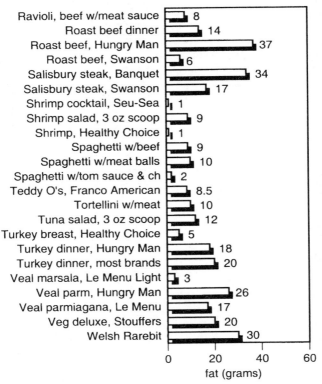

## COMBINED AND FROZEN FOODS*,
### Part 4

| Food | fat (grams) |
|------|-------------|
| Ravioli, beef w/meat sauce | 8 |
| Roast beef dinner | 14 |
| Roast beef, Hungry Man | 37 |
| Roast beef, Swanson | 6 |
| Salisbury steak, Banquet | 34 |
| Salisbury steak, Swanson | 17 |
| Shrimp cocktail, Seu-Sea | 1 |
| Shrimp salad, 3 oz scoop | 9 |
| Shrimp, Healthy Choice | 1 |
| Spaghetti w/beef | 9 |
| Spaghetti w/meat balls | 10 |
| Spaghetti w/tom sauce & ch | 2 |
| Teddy O's, Franco American | 8.5 |
| Tortellini w/meat | 10 |
| Tuna salad, 3 oz scoop | 12 |
| Turkey breast, Healthy Choice | 5 |
| Turkey dinner, Hungry Man | 18 |
| Turkey dinner, most brands | 20 |
| Veal marsala, Le Menu Light | 3 |
| Veal parm, Hungry Man | 26 |
| Veal parmiagana, Le Menu | 17 |
| Veg deluxe, Stouffers | 20 |
| Welsh Rarebit | 30 |

fat (grams)

\* Counts are based on average-size servings as indicated
on package. Adjust count to reflect amount consumed.

## Dairy: CHEESE (HARD & SEMI-SOFT)*

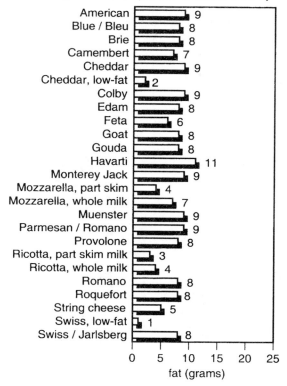

| Cheese | fat (grams) |
|--------|-------------|
| American | 9 |
| Blue / Bleu | 8 |
| Brie | 8 |
| Camembert | 7 |
| Cheddar | 9 |
| Cheddar, low-fat | 2 |
| Colby | 9 |
| Edam | 8 |
| Feta | 6 |
| Goat | 8 |
| Gouda | 8 |
| Havarti | 11 |
| Monterey Jack | 9 |
| Mozzarella, part skim | 4 |
| Mozzarella, whole milk | 7 |
| Muenster | 9 |
| Parmesan / Romano | 9 |
| Provolone | 8 |
| Ricotta, part skim milk | 3 |
| Ricotta, whole milk | 4 |
| Romano | 8 |
| Roquefort | 8 |
| String cheese | 5 |
| Swiss, low-fat | 1 |
| Swiss / Jarlsberg | 8 |

fat (grams): 0  5  10  15  20  25

\* Counts are based on one-ounce servings. Adjust count
to reflect amount consumed.

## Dairy: CHEESES (SOFT), CREAMS & SUBSTITUTES*

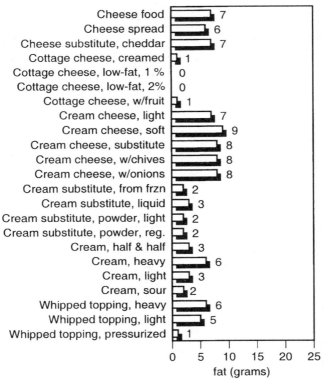

| | fat (grams) |
|---|---|
| Cheese food | 7 |
| Cheese spread | 6 |
| Cheese substitute, cheddar | 7 |
| Cottage cheese, creamed | 1 |
| Cottage cheese, low-fat, 1 % | 0 |
| Cottage cheese, low-fat, 2% | 0 |
| Cottage cheese, w/fruit | 1 |
| Cream cheese, light | 7 |
| Cream cheese, soft | 9 |
| Cream cheese, substitute | 8 |
| Cream cheese, w/chives | 8 |
| Cream cheese, w/onions | 8 |
| Cream substitute, from frzn | 2 |
| Cream substitute, liquid | 3 |
| Cream substitute, powder, light | 2 |
| Cream substitute, powder, reg. | 2 |
| Cream, half & half | 3 |
| Cream, heavy | 6 |
| Cream, light | 3 |
| Cream, sour | 2 |
| Whipped topping, heavy | 6 |
| Whipped topping, light | 5 |
| Whipped topping, pressurized | 1 |

* Counts are based on one-ounce servings of soft cheese
or one tablespoon of cream or whipped topping.

## Dairy: EGGS, MILK, YOGURT & SHAKES*

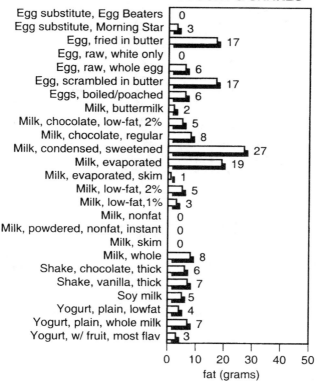

| Food | fat (grams) |
|---|---|
| Egg substitute, Egg Beaters | 0 |
| Egg substitute, Morning Star | 3 |
| Egg, fried in butter | 17 |
| Egg, raw, white only | 0 |
| Egg, raw, whole egg | 6 |
| Egg, scrambled in butter | 17 |
| Eggs, boiled/poached | 6 |
| Milk, buttermilk | 2 |
| Milk, chocolate, low-fat, 2% | 5 |
| Milk, chocolate, regular | 8 |
| Milk, condensed, sweetened | 27 |
| Milk, evaporated | 19 |
| Milk, evaporated, skim | 1 |
| Milk, low-fat, 2% | 5 |
| Milk, low-fat,1% | 3 |
| Milk, nonfat | 0 |
| Milk, powdered, nonfat, instant | 0 |
| Milk, skim | 0 |
| Milk, whole | 8 |
| Shake, chocolate, thick | 6 |
| Shake, vanilla, thick | 7 |
| Soy milk | 5 |
| Yogurt, plain, lowfat | 4 |
| Yogurt, plain, whole milk | 7 |
| Yogurt, w/ fruit, most flav | 3 |

fat (grams) — 0  10  20  30  40  50

* Counts based on one egg or equivalent egg substitute or 8 fluid ounces of milk, yogurt, or shake.

**Dining Out: ASIAN\***

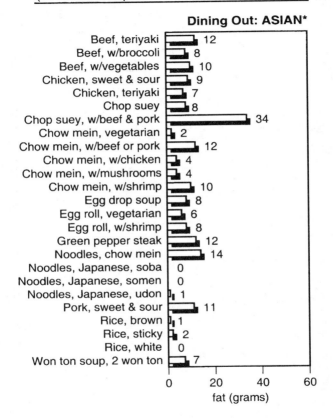

| | |
|---|---|
| Beef, teriyaki | 12 |
| Beef, w/broccoli | 8 |
| Beef, w/vegetables | 10 |
| Chicken, sweet & sour | 9 |
| Chicken, teriyaki | 7 |
| Chop suey | 8 |
| Chop suey, w/beef & pork | 34 |
| Chow mein, vegetarian | 2 |
| Chow mein, w/beef or pork | 12 |
| Chow mein, w/chicken | 4 |
| Chow mein, w/mushrooms | 4 |
| Chow mein, w/shrimp | 10 |
| Egg drop soup | 8 |
| Egg roll, vegetarian | 6 |
| Egg roll, w/shrimp | 8 |
| Green pepper steak | 12 |
| Noodles, chow mein | 14 |
| Noodles, Japanese, soba | 0 |
| Noodles, Japanese, somen | 0 |
| Noodles, Japanese, udon | 1 |
| Pork, sweet & sour | 11 |
| Rice, brown | 1 |
| Rice, sticky | 2 |
| Rice, white | 0 |
| Won ton soup, 2 won ton | 7 |

0    20    40    60
fat (grams)

\* Counts based on average-sized servings (for main dishes,
1 1/2 - 2 cups).  Counts for main dishes include rice.

24

## Dining Out: DELICATESSEN*

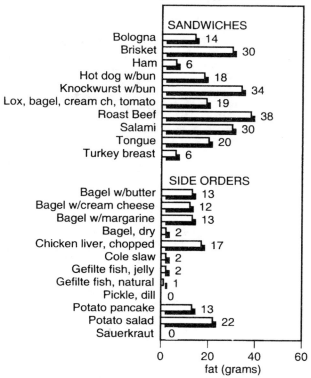

SANDWICHES

| | fat (grams) |
|---|---|
| Bologna | 14 |
| Brisket | 30 |
| Ham | 6 |
| Hot dog w/bun | 18 |
| Knockwurst w/bun | 34 |
| Lox, bagel, cream ch, tomato | 19 |
| Roast Beef | 38 |
| Salami | 30 |
| Tongue | 20 |
| Turkey breast | 6 |

SIDE ORDERS

| | fat (grams) |
|---|---|
| Bagel w/butter | 13 |
| Bagel w/cream cheese | 12 |
| Bagel w/margarine | 13 |
| Bagel, dry | 2 |
| Chicken liver, chopped | 17 |
| Cole slaw | 2 |
| Gefilte fish, jelly | 2 |
| Gefilte fish, natural | 1 |
| Pickle, dill | 0 |
| Potato pancake | 13 |
| Potato salad | 22 |
| Sauerkraut | 0 |

fat (grams)

* Unless otherwise indicated, counts based on average-size servings or sandwiches. Sandwich counts assume white or rye bread.

25

## Dining Out: FRENCH AND OTHER INTERNATIONAL DISHES*

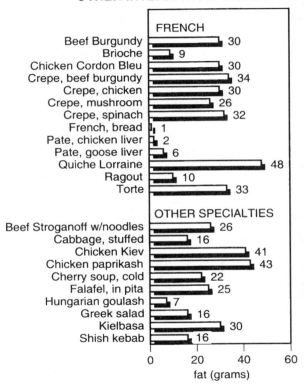

**FRENCH**

| Dish | fat (grams) |
|------|-------------|
| Beef Burgundy | 30 |
| Brioche | 9 |
| Chicken Cordon Bleu | 30 |
| Crepe, beef burgundy | 34 |
| Crepe, chicken | 30 |
| Crepe, mushroom | 26 |
| Crepe, spinach | 32 |
| French, bread | 1 |
| Pate, chicken liver | 2 |
| Pate, goose liver | 6 |
| Quiche Lorraine | 48 |
| Ragout | 10 |
| Torte | 33 |

**OTHER SPECIALTIES**

| Dish | fat (grams) |
|------|-------------|
| Beef Stroganoff w/noodles | 26 |
| Cabbage, stuffed | 16 |
| Chicken Kiev | 41 |
| Chicken paprikash | 43 |
| Cherry soup, cold | 22 |
| Falafel, in pita | 25 |
| Hungarian goulash | 7 |
| Greek salad | 16 |
| Kielbasa | 30 |
| Shish kebab | 16 |

fat (grams)

\* Counts based on average-sized servings (for main dishes, 1 1/2 - 2 cups).

Alphabetical Chart
(for Hi-Low Comparison Charts, see pages 83 - 164)

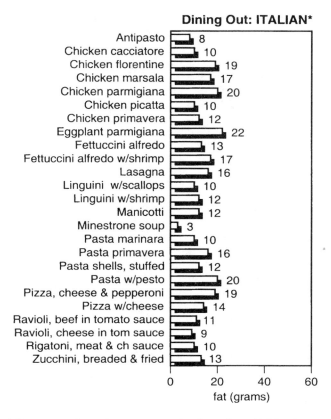

**Dining Out: ITALIAN\***

| Item | fat (grams) |
|---|---|
| Antipasto | 8 |
| Chicken cacciatore | 10 |
| Chicken florentine | 19 |
| Chicken marsala | 17 |
| Chicken parmigiana | 20 |
| Chicken picatta | 10 |
| Chicken primavera | 12 |
| Eggplant parmigiana | 22 |
| Fettuccini alfredo | 13 |
| Fettuccini alfredo w/shrimp | 17 |
| Lasagna | 16 |
| Linguini w/scallops | 10 |
| Linguini w/shrimp | 12 |
| Manicotti | 12 |
| Minestrone soup | 3 |
| Pasta marinara | 10 |
| Pasta primavera | 16 |
| Pasta shells, stuffed | 12 |
| Pasta w/pesto | 20 |
| Pizza, cheese & pepperoni | 19 |
| Pizza w/cheese | 14 |
| Ravioli, beef in tomato sauce | 11 |
| Ravioli, cheese in tom sauce | 9 |
| Rigatoni, meat & ch sauce | 10 |
| Zucchini, breaded & fried | 13 |

fat (grams)

\* Counts are based on average-sized servings (1 1/2 - 2 cups); for pizza, on 1/6 medium or 1/8 large pizza).

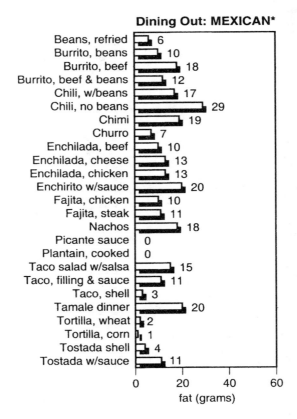

**Dining Out: MEXICAN\***

| Food | fat (grams) |
|---|---|
| Beans, refried | 6 |
| Burrito, beans | 10 |
| Burrito, beef | 18 |
| Burrito, beef & beans | 12 |
| Chili, w/beans | 17 |
| Chili, no beans | 29 |
| Chimi | 19 |
| Churro | 7 |
| Enchilada, beef | 10 |
| Enchilada, cheese | 13 |
| Enchilada, chicken | 13 |
| Enchirito w/sauce | 20 |
| Fajita, chicken | 10 |
| Fajita, steak | 11 |
| Nachos | 18 |
| Picante sauce | 0 |
| Plantain, cooked | 0 |
| Taco salad w/salsa | 15 |
| Taco, filling & sauce | 11 |
| Taco, shell | 3 |
| Tamale dinner | 20 |
| Tortilla, wheat | 2 |
| Tortilla, corn | 1 |
| Tostada shell | 4 |
| Tostada w/sauce | 11 |

\* Counts based on average-sized servings (for main dishes, 1 1/2 - 2 cups).

## Fast Food: ARBY'S*

| Item | fat (grams) |
|---|---|
| Baked potato, broc & cheddar | 20 |
| Baked potato, deluxe | 36 |
| Baked potato, plain | 0 |
| Baked potato, sour cream | 24 |
| French fries, curly | 15 |
| French fries, curly w/cheddar | 18 |
| Sandwich, Arby-Q | 18 |
| Sandwich, bacon'n ch, deluxe | 34 |
| Sandwich, chick club, roasted | 31 |
| Sandwich, chicken, BBQ | 13 |
| Sandwich, chicken, breaded | 28 |
| Sandwich, chicken, Cordon Bl | 33 |
| Sandwich, chicken, grilled | 20 |
| Sandwich, chicken, Santa Fe | 22 |
| Sandwich, fish fillet | 27 |
| Sandwich, French dip | 22 |
| Sandwich, ham 'n swiss, hot | 23 |
| Sandwich, ham'n cheese melt | 13 |
| Sandwich, Italian sub | 36 |
| Sandwich, Philly beef'n swiss | 47 |
| Sandwich, roast beef deluxe | 10 |
| Sandwich, roast beef sub | 42 |
| Sandwich, roast beef, giant | 28 |
| Sandwich, triple cheese melt | 45 |
| Sandwich, turkey club | 27 |

0     25     50     75     100
fat (grams)

\* Unless otherwise indicated, counts are based on average-
size servings.

**Fast Food: BOSTON MARKET***

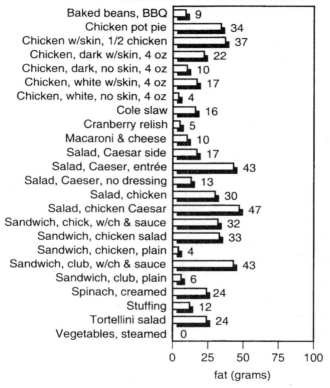

| | fat (grams) |
|---|---|
| Baked beans, BBQ | 9 |
| Chicken pot pie | 34 |
| Chicken w/skin, 1/2 chicken | 37 |
| Chicken, dark w/skin, 4 oz | 22 |
| Chicken, dark, no skin, 4 oz | 10 |
| Chicken, white w/skin, 4 oz | 17 |
| Chicken, white, no skin, 4 oz | 4 |
| Cole slaw | 16 |
| Cranberry relish | 5 |
| Macaroni & cheese | 10 |
| Salad, Caesar side | 17 |
| Salad, Caeser, entrée | 43 |
| Salad, Caeser, no dressing | 13 |
| Salad, chicken | 30 |
| Salad, chicken Caesar | 47 |
| Sandwich, chick, w/ch & sauce | 32 |
| Sandwich, chicken salad | 33 |
| Sandwich, chicken, plain | 4 |
| Sandwich, club, w/ch & sauce | 43 |
| Sandwich, club, plain | 6 |
| Spinach, creamed | 24 |
| Stuffing | 12 |
| Tortellini salad | 24 |
| Vegetables, steamed | 0 |

* Unless otherwise indicated, counts are based on average-size servings.

## Fast Food: BURGER KING*

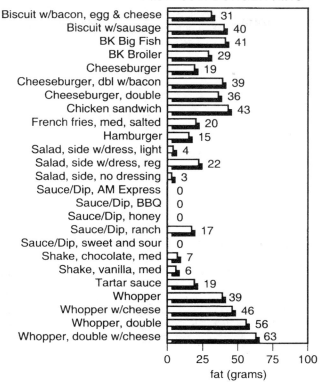

| Item | fat (grams) |
|---|---|
| Biscuit w/bacon, egg & cheese | 31 |
| Biscuit w/sausage | 40 |
| BK Big Fish | 41 |
| BK Broiler | 29 |
| Cheeseburger | 19 |
| Cheeseburger, dbl w/bacon | 39 |
| Cheeseburger, double | 36 |
| Chicken sandwich | 43 |
| French fries, med, salted | 20 |
| Hamburger | 15 |
| Salad, side w/dress, light | 4 |
| Salad, side w/dress, reg | 22 |
| Salad, side, no dressing | 3 |
| Sauce/Dip, AM Express | 0 |
| Sauce/Dip, BBQ | 0 |
| Sauce/Dip, honey | 0 |
| Sauce/Dip, ranch | 17 |
| Sauce/Dip, sweet and sour | 0 |
| Shake, chocolate, med | 7 |
| Shake, vanilla, med | 6 |
| Tartar sauce | 19 |
| Whopper | 39 |
| Whopper w/cheese | 46 |
| Whopper, double | 56 |
| Whopper, double w/cheese | 63 |

fat (grams)

* Unless otherwise indicated, counts are based on average-
size servings.

**Fast Food: HARDEE'S***

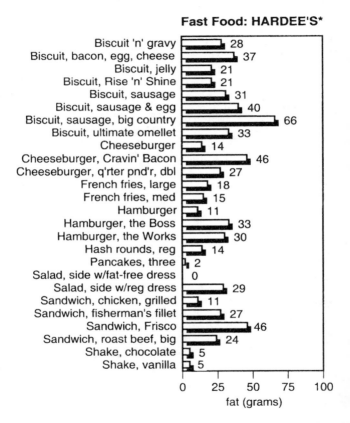

| Item | fat (grams) |
|---|---|
| Biscuit 'n' gravy | 28 |
| Biscuit, bacon, egg, cheese | 37 |
| Biscuit, jelly | 21 |
| Biscuit, Rise 'n' Shine | 21 |
| Biscuit, sausage | 31 |
| Biscuit, sausage & egg | 40 |
| Biscuit, sausage, big country | 66 |
| Biscuit, ultimate omellet | 33 |
| Cheeseburger | 14 |
| Cheeseburger, Cravin' Bacon | 46 |
| Cheeseburger, q'rter pnd'r, dbl | 27 |
| French fries, large | 18 |
| French fries, med | 15 |
| Hamburger | 11 |
| Hamburger, the Boss | 33 |
| Hamburger, the Works | 30 |
| Hash rounds, reg | 14 |
| Pancakes, three | 2 |
| Salad, side w/fat-free dress | 0 |
| Salad, side w/reg dress | 29 |
| Sandwich, chicken, grilled | 11 |
| Sandwich, fisherman's fillet | 27 |
| Sandwich, Frisco | 46 |
| Sandwich, roast beef, big | 24 |
| Shake, chocolate | 5 |
| Shake, vanilla | 5 |

fat (grams)

\* Unless otherwise indicated, counts are based on average-size servings.

## Fast Food: JACK IN THE BOX*

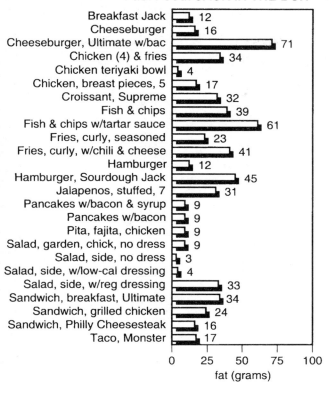

| Item | fat (grams) |
|------|-------------|
| Breakfast Jack | 12 |
| Cheeseburger | 16 |
| Cheeseburger, Ultimate w/bac | 71 |
| Chicken (4) & fries | 34 |
| Chicken teriyaki bowl | 4 |
| Chicken, breast pieces, 5 | 17 |
| Croissant, Supreme | 32 |
| Fish & chips | 39 |
| Fish & chips w/tartar sauce | 61 |
| Fries, curly, seasoned | 23 |
| Fries, curly, w/chili & cheese | 41 |
| Hamburger | 12 |
| Hamburger, Sourdough Jack | 45 |
| Jalapenos, stuffed, 7 | 31 |
| Pancakes w/bacon & syrup | 9 |
| Pancakes w/bacon | 9 |
| Pita, fajita, chicken | 9 |
| Salad, garden, chick, no dress | 9 |
| Salad, side, no dress | 3 |
| Salad, side, w/low-cal dressing | 4 |
| Salad, side, w/reg dressing | 33 |
| Sandwich, breakfast, Ultimate | 34 |
| Sandwich, grilled chicken | 24 |
| Sandwich, Philly Cheesesteak | 16 |
| Taco, Monster | 17 |

fat (grams)

\* Unless otherwise indicated, counts are based on average-size servings.

**Fast Food: KFC\***

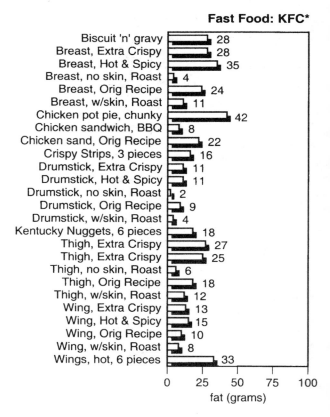

| Item | fat (grams) |
|------|-------------|
| Biscuit 'n' gravy | 28 |
| Breast, Extra Crispy | 28 |
| Breast, Hot & Spicy | 35 |
| Breast, no skin, Roast | 4 |
| Breast, Orig Recipe | 24 |
| Breast, w/skin, Roast | 11 |
| Chicken pot pie, chunky | 42 |
| Chicken sandwich, BBQ | 8 |
| Chicken sand, Orig Recipe | 22 |
| Crispy Strips, 3 pieces | 16 |
| Drumstick, Extra Crispy | 11 |
| Drumstick, Hot & Spicy | 11 |
| Drumstick, no skin, Roast | 2 |
| Drumstick, Orig Recipe | 9 |
| Drumstick, w/skin, Roast | 4 |
| Kentucky Nuggets, 6 pieces | 18 |
| Thigh, Extra Crispy | 27 |
| Thigh, Extra Crispy | 25 |
| Thigh, no skin, Roast | 6 |
| Thigh, Orig Recipe | 18 |
| Thigh, w/skin, Roast | 12 |
| Wing, Extra Crispy | 13 |
| Wing, Hot & Spicy | 15 |
| Wing, Orig Recipe | 10 |
| Wing, w/skin, Roast | 8 |
| Wings, hot, 6 pieces | 33 |

\* Unless otherwise indicated, counts are based on average-size servings.

34

**Fast Food:  MC DONALD'S\***

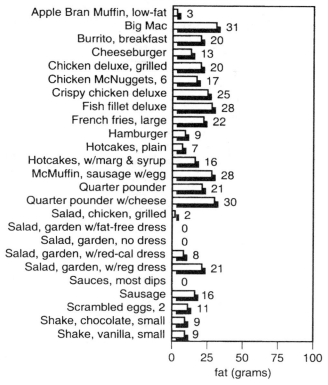

| Item | fat (grams) |
|------|-------------|
| Apple Bran Muffin, low-fat | 3 |
| Big Mac | 31 |
| Burrito, breakfast | 20 |
| Cheeseburger | 13 |
| Chicken deluxe, grilled | 20 |
| Chicken McNuggets, 6 | 17 |
| Crispy chicken deluxe | 25 |
| Fish fillet deluxe | 28 |
| French fries, large | 22 |
| Hamburger | 9 |
| Hotcakes, plain | 7 |
| Hotcakes, w/marg & syrup | 16 |
| McMuffin, sausage w/egg | 28 |
| Quarter pounder | 21 |
| Quarter pounder w/cheese | 30 |
| Salad, chicken, grilled | 2 |
| Salad, garden w/fat-free dress | 0 |
| Salad, garden, no dress | 0 |
| Salad, garden, w/red-cal dress | 8 |
| Salad, garden, w/reg dress | 21 |
| Sauces, most dips | 0 |
| Sausage | 16 |
| Scrambled eggs, 2 | 11 |
| Shake, chocolate, small | 9 |
| Shake, vanilla, small | 9 |

fat (grams)

\* Unless otherwise indicated, counts are based on average-size servings.

35

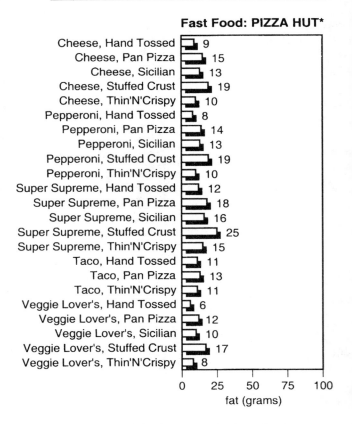

## Alphabetical Chart
(for Hi-Low Comparison Charts, see pages 83 - 164)

### Fast Food: PIZZA HUT*

| Item | fat (grams) |
|---|---|
| Cheese, Hand Tossed | 9 |
| Cheese, Pan Pizza | 15 |
| Cheese, Sicilian | 13 |
| Cheese, Stuffed Crust | 19 |
| Cheese, Thin'N'Crispy | 10 |
| Pepperoni, Hand Tossed | 8 |
| Pepperoni, Pan Pizza | 14 |
| Pepperoni, Sicilian | 13 |
| Pepperoni, Stuffed Crust | 19 |
| Pepperoni, Thin'N'Crispy | 10 |
| Super Supreme, Hand Tossed | 12 |
| Super Supreme, Pan Pizza | 18 |
| Super Supreme, Sicilian | 16 |
| Super Supreme, Stuffed Crust | 25 |
| Super Supreme, Thin'N'Crispy | 15 |
| Taco, Hand Tossed | 11 |
| Taco, Pan Pizza | 13 |
| Taco, Thin'N'Crispy | 11 |
| Veggie Lover's, Hand Tossed | 6 |
| Veggie Lover's, Pan Pizza | 12 |
| Veggie Lover's, Sicilian | 10 |
| Veggie Lover's, Stuffed Crust | 17 |
| Veggie Lover's, Thin'N'Crispy | 8 |

fat (grams) — 0, 25, 50, 75, 100

\* Unless otherwise indicated, counts are based on average-size servings.

**Fast Food: SUBWAY***

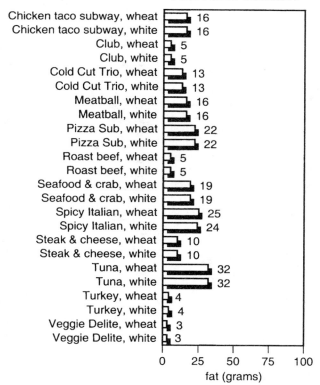

| | fat (grams) |
|---|---|
| Chicken taco subway, wheat | 16 |
| Chicken taco subway, white | 16 |
| Club, wheat | 5 |
| Club, white | 5 |
| Cold Cut Trio, wheat | 13 |
| Cold Cut Trio, white | 13 |
| Meatball, wheat | 16 |
| Meatball, white | 16 |
| Pizza Sub, wheat | 22 |
| Pizza Sub, white | 22 |
| Roast beef, wheat | 5 |
| Roast beef, white | 5 |
| Seafood & crab, wheat | 19 |
| Seafood & crab, white | 19 |
| Spicy Italian, wheat | 25 |
| Spicy Italian, white | 24 |
| Steak & cheese, wheat | 10 |
| Steak & cheese, white | 10 |
| Tuna, wheat | 32 |
| Tuna, white | 32 |
| Turkey, wheat | 4 |
| Turkey, white | 4 |
| Veggie Delite, wheat | 3 |
| Veggie Delite, white | 3 |

\* Unless otherwise indicated, counts are based on average-size servings.

**Fast Food: TACO BELL\***

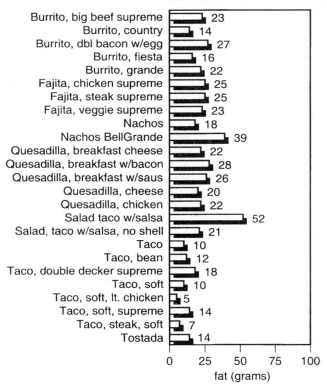

| | fat (grams) |
|---|---|
| Burrito, big beef supreme | 23 |
| Burrito, country | 14 |
| Burrito, dbl bacon w/egg | 27 |
| Burrito, fiesta | 16 |
| Burrito, grande | 22 |
| Fajita, chicken supreme | 25 |
| Fajita, steak supreme | 25 |
| Fajita, veggie supreme | 23 |
| Nachos | 18 |
| Nachos BellGrande | 39 |
| Quesadilla, breakfast cheese | 22 |
| Quesadilla, breakfast w/bacon | 28 |
| Quesadilla, breakfast w/saus | 26 |
| Quesadilla, cheese | 20 |
| Quesadilla, chicken | 22 |
| Salad taco w/salsa | 52 |
| Salad, taco w/salsa, no shell | 21 |
| Taco | 10 |
| Taco, bean | 12 |
| Taco, double decker supreme | 18 |
| Taco, soft | 10 |
| Taco, soft, lt. chicken | 5 |
| Taco, soft, supreme | 14 |
| Taco, steak, soft | 7 |
| Tostada | 14 |

\* Unless otherwise indicated, counts are based on average-size servings.

38

**Fast Food: WENDY'S***

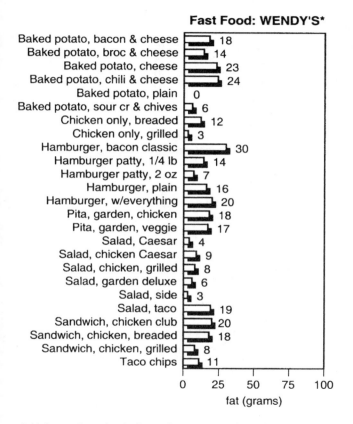

| | fat (grams) |
|---|---|
| Baked potato, bacon & cheese | 18 |
| Baked potato, broc & cheese | 14 |
| Baked potato, cheese | 23 |
| Baked potato, chili & cheese | 24 |
| Baked potato, plain | 0 |
| Baked potato, sour cr & chives | 6 |
| Chicken only, breaded | 12 |
| Chicken only, grilled | 3 |
| Hamburger, bacon classic | 30 |
| Hamburger patty, 1/4 lb | 14 |
| Hamburger patty, 2 oz | 7 |
| Hamburger, plain | 16 |
| Hamburger, w/everything | 20 |
| Pita, garden, chicken | 18 |
| Pita, garden, veggie | 17 |
| Salad, Caesar | 4 |
| Salad, chicken Caesar | 9 |
| Salad, chicken, grilled | 8 |
| Salad, garden deluxe | 6 |
| Salad, side | 3 |
| Salad, taco | 19 |
| Sandwich, chicken club | 20 |
| Sandwich, chicken, breaded | 18 |
| Sandwich, chicken, grilled | 8 |
| Taco chips | 11 |

fat (grams)

* Unless otherwise indicated, counts are based on average-
size servings.

## Fruits: FRESH & DRIED FRUITS AND JUICES *, Part 1

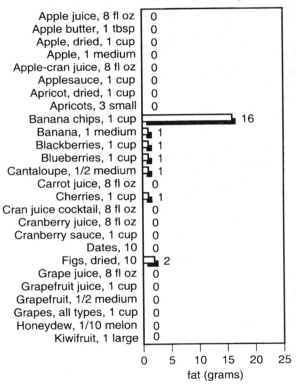

| | fat (grams) |
|---|---|
| Apple juice, 8 fl oz | 0 |
| Apple butter, 1 tbsp | 0 |
| Apple, dried, 1 cup | 0 |
| Apple, 1 medium | 0 |
| Apple-cran juice, 8 fl oz | 0 |
| Applesauce, 1 cup | 0 |
| Apricot, dried, 1 cup | 0 |
| Apricots, 3 small | 0 |
| Banana chips, 1 cup | 16 |
| Banana, 1 medium | 1 |
| Blackberries, 1 cup | 1 |
| Blueberries, 1 cup | 1 |
| Cantaloupe, 1/2 medium | 1 |
| Carrot juice, 8 fl oz | 0 |
| Cherries, 1 cup | 1 |
| Cran juice cocktail, 8 fl oz | 0 |
| Cranberry juice, 8 fl oz | 0 |
| Cranberry sauce, 1 cup | 0 |
| Dates, 10 | 0 |
| Figs, dried, 10 | 2 |
| Grape juice, 8 fl oz | 0 |
| Grapefruit juice, 1 cup | 0 |
| Grapefruit, 1/2 medium | 0 |
| Grapes, all types, 1 cup | 0 |
| Honeydew, 1/10 melon | 0 |
| Kiwifruit, 1 large | 0 |

* Unless otherwise indicated, counts are based on whole, fresh fruits.

## Fruits: FRESH & DRIED FRUITS
## AND  JUICES *, Part 2

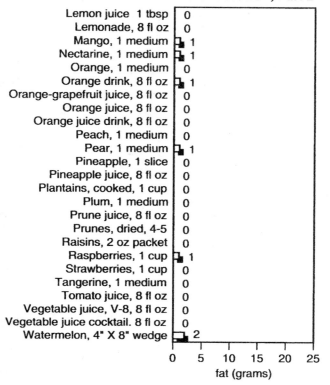

| | fat (grams) |
|---|---|
| Lemon juice  1 tbsp | 0 |
| Lemonade, 8 fl oz | 0 |
| Mango, 1 medium | 1 |
| Nectarine, 1 medium | 1 |
| Orange, 1 medium | 0 |
| Orange drink, 8 fl oz | 1 |
| Orange-grapefruit juice, 8 fl oz | 0 |
| Orange juice, 8 fl oz | 0 |
| Orange juice drink, 8 fl oz | 0 |
| Peach, 1 medium | 0 |
| Pear, 1 medium | 1 |
| Pineapple, 1 slice | 0 |
| Pineapple juice, 8 fl oz | 0 |
| Plantains, cooked, 1 cup | 0 |
| Plum, 1 medium | 0 |
| Prune juice, 8 fl oz | 0 |
| Prunes, dried, 4-5 | 0 |
| Raisins, 2 oz packet | 0 |
| Raspberries, 1 cup | 1 |
| Strawberries, 1 cup | 0 |
| Tangerine, 1 medium | 0 |
| Tomato juice, 8 fl oz | 0 |
| Vegetable juice, V-8, 8 fl oz | 0 |
| Vegetable juice cocktail. 8 fl oz | 0 |
| Watermelon, 4" X 8" wedge | 2 |

0    5    10    15    20    25
fat (grams)

* Unless otherwise indicated, counts are based on whole,
  fresh fruits.

41

## GRAVIES, SAUCES & DIPS*

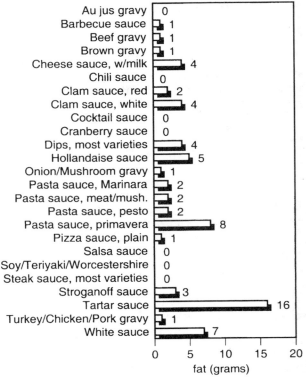

| Sauce | fat (grams) |
|---|---|
| Au jus gravy | 0 |
| Barbecue sauce | 1 |
| Beef gravy | 1 |
| Brown gravy | 1 |
| Cheese sauce, w/milk | 4 |
| Chili sauce | 0 |
| Clam sauce, red | 2 |
| Clam sauce, white | 4 |
| Cocktail sauce | 0 |
| Cranberry sauce | 0 |
| Dips, most varieties | 4 |
| Hollandaise sauce | 5 |
| Onion/Mushroom gravy | 1 |
| Pasta sauce, Marinara | 2 |
| Pasta sauce, meat/mush. | 2 |
| Pasta sauce, pesto | 2 |
| Pasta sauce, primavera | 8 |
| Pizza sauce, plain | 1 |
| Salsa sauce | 0 |
| Soy/Teriyaki/Worcestershire | 0 |
| Steak sauce, most varieties | 0 |
| Stroganoff sauce | 3 |
| Tartar sauce | 16 |
| Turkey/Chicken/Pork gravy | 1 |
| White sauce | 7 |

*Counts are based on one-quarter cup servings.

**MEATS\*, Part 1**

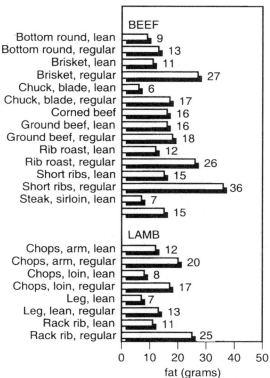

BEEF

| | fat (grams) |
|---|---|
| Bottom round, lean | 9 |
| Bottom round, regular | 13 |
| Brisket, lean | 11 |
| Brisket, regular | 27 |
| Chuck, blade, lean | 6 |
| Chuck, blade, regular | 17 |
| Corned beef | 16 |
| Ground beef, lean | 16 |
| Ground beef, regular | 18 |
| Rib roast, lean | 12 |
| Rib roast, regular | 26 |
| Short ribs, lean | 15 |
| Short ribs, regular | 36 |
| Steak, sirloin, lean | 7 |
| | 15 |

LAMB

| | fat (grams) |
|---|---|
| Chops, arm, lean | 12 |
| Chops, arm, regular | 20 |
| Chops, loin, lean | 8 |
| Chops, loin, regular | 17 |
| Leg, lean | 7 |
| Leg, lean, regular | 13 |
| Rack rib, lean | 11 |
| Rack rib, regular | 25 |

fat (grams)

\* Counts are based on 3-ounce servings.

43

**MEATS\*, Part 2**

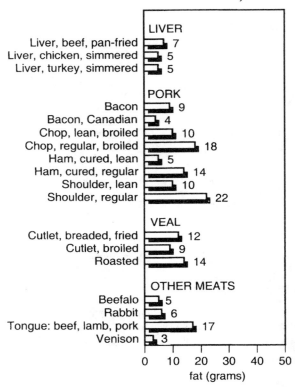

LIVER

| | |
|---|---|
| Liver, beef, pan-fried | 7 |
| Liver, chicken, simmered | 5 |
| Liver, turkey, simmered | 5 |

PORK

| | |
|---|---|
| Bacon | 9 |
| Bacon, Canadian | 4 |
| Chop, lean, broiled | 10 |
| Chop, regular, broiled | 18 |
| Ham, cured, lean | 5 |
| Ham, cured, regular | 14 |
| Shoulder, lean | 10 |
| Shoulder, regular | 22 |

VEAL

| | |
|---|---|
| Cutlet, breaded, fried | 12 |
| Cutlet, broiled | 9 |
| Roasted | 14 |

OTHER MEATS

| | |
|---|---|
| Beefalo | 5 |
| Rabbit | 6 |
| Tongue: beef, lamb, pork | 17 |
| Venison | 3 |

0   10   20   30   40   50

fat (grams)

\* Counts are based on 3-ounce servings.

44

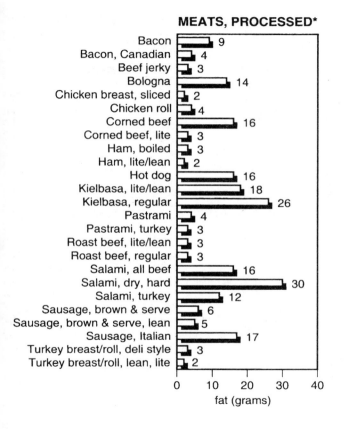

**MEATS, PROCESSED***

| Item | fat (grams) |
|------|-------------|
| Bacon | 9 |
| Bacon, Canadian | 4 |
| Beef jerky | 3 |
| Bologna | 14 |
| Chicken breast, sliced | 2 |
| Chicken roll | 4 |
| Corned beef | 16 |
| Corned beef, lite | 3 |
| Ham, boiled | 3 |
| Ham, lite/lean | 2 |
| Hot dog | 16 |
| Kielbasa, lite/lean | 18 |
| Kielbasa, regular | 26 |
| Pastrami | 4 |
| Pastrami, turkey | 3 |
| Roast beef, lite/lean | 3 |
| Roast beef, regular | 3 |
| Salami, all beef | 16 |
| Salami, dry, hard | 30 |
| Salami, turkey | 12 |
| Sausage, brown & serve | 6 |
| Sausage, brown & serve, lean | 5 |
| Sausage, Italian | 17 |
| Turkey breast/roll, deli style | 3 |
| Turkey breast/roll, lean, lite | 2 |

fat (grams)

* Counts are based on 3-ounce servings.

**Medications: COUGH DROPS & SYRUPS\***

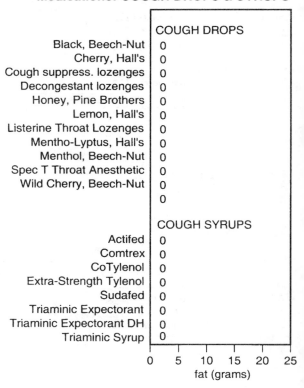

| | COUGH DROPS |
|---|---|
| Black, Beech-Nut | 0 |
| Cherry, Hall's | 0 |
| Cough suppress. lozenges | 0 |
| Decongestant lozenges | 0 |
| Honey, Pine Brothers | 0 |
| Lemon, Hall's | 0 |
| Listerine Throat Lozenges | 0 |
| Mentho-Lyptus, Hall's | 0 |
| Menthol, Beech-Nut | 0 |
| Spec T Throat Anesthetic | 0 |
| Wild Cherry, Beech-Nut | 0 |
| | 0 |
| | COUGH SYRUPS |
| Actifed | 0 |
| Comtrex | 0 |
| CoTylenol | 0 |
| Extra-Strength Tylenol | 0 |
| Sudafed | 0 |
| Triaminic Expectorant | 0 |
| Triaminic Expectorant DH | 0 |
| Triaminic Syrup | 0 |

0    5    10    15    20    25
fat (grams)

\* Counts are based on one cough drop or on recommended
doses for adults.

## Medications: OVER-THE-COUNTER REMEDIES & VITAMINS AND MINERALS*

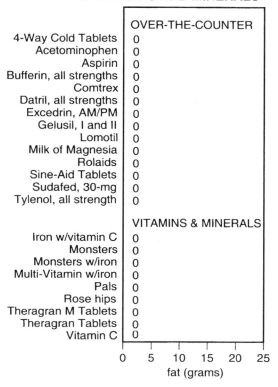

| | OVER-THE-COUNTER |
|---|---|
| 4-Way Cold Tablets | 0 |
| Acetominophen | 0 |
| Aspirin | 0 |
| Bufferin, all strengths | 0 |
| Comtrex | 0 |
| Datril, all strengths | 0 |
| Excedrin, AM/PM | 0 |
| Gelusil, I and II | 0 |
| Lomotil | 0 |
| Milk of Magnesia | 0 |
| Rolaids | 0 |
| Sine-Aid Tablets | 0 |
| Sudafed, 30-mg | 0 |
| Tylenol, all strength | 0 |

| | VITAMINS & MINERALS |
|---|---|
| Iron w/vitamin C | 0 |
| Monsters | 0 |
| Monsters w/iron | 0 |
| Multi-Vitamin w/iron | 0 |
| Pals | 0 |
| Rose hips | 0 |
| Theragran M Tablets | 0 |
| Theragran Tablets | 0 |
| Vitamin C | 0 |

```
0    5    10   15   20   25
          fat (grams)
```

* Counts are based on recommended doses for adults.

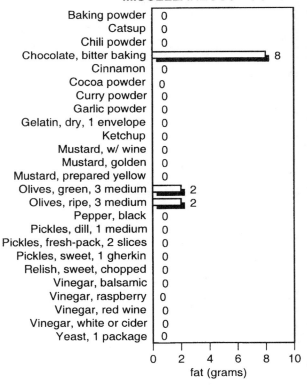

**MISCELLANEOUS FOODS***

| Food | fat (grams) |
|------|-------------|
| Baking powder | 0 |
| Catsup | 0 |
| Chili powder | 0 |
| Chocolate, bitter baking | 8 |
| Cinnamon | 0 |
| Cocoa powder | 0 |
| Curry powder | 0 |
| Garlic powder | 0 |
| Gelatin, dry, 1 envelope | 0 |
| Ketchup | 0 |
| Mustard, w/ wine | 0 |
| Mustard, golden | 0 |
| Mustard, prepared yellow | 0 |
| Olives, green, 3 medium | 2 |
| Olives, ripe, 3 medium | 2 |
| Pepper, black | 0 |
| Pickles, dill, 1 medium | 0 |
| Pickles, fresh-pack, 2 slices | 0 |
| Pickles, sweet, 1 gherkin | 0 |
| Relish, sweet, chopped | 0 |
| Vinegar, balsamic | 0 |
| Vinegar, raspberry | 0 |
| Vinegar, red wine | 0 |
| Vinegar, white or cider | 0 |
| Yeast, 1 package | 0 |

\* Unless otherwise indicated, counts are based on
a one-tablespoon serving.

## NUTS, BEANS AND SEEDS*: Part 1

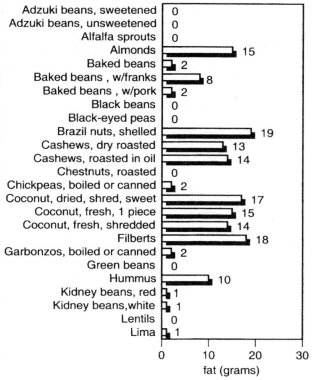

| | fat (grams) |
|---|---|
| Adzuki beans, sweetened | 0 |
| Adzuki beans, unsweetened | 0 |
| Alfalfa sprouts | 0 |
| Almonds | 15 |
| Baked beans | 2 |
| Baked beans , w/franks | 8 |
| Baked beans , w/pork | 2 |
| Black beans | 0 |
| Black-eyed peas | 0 |
| Brazil nuts, shelled | 19 |
| Cashews, dry roasted | 13 |
| Cashews, roasted in oil | 14 |
| Chestnuts, roasted | 0 |
| Chickpeas, boiled or canned | 2 |
| Coconut, dried, shred, sweet | 17 |
| Coconut, fresh, 1 piece | 15 |
| Coconut, fresh, shredded | 14 |
| Filberts | 18 |
| Garbonzos, boiled or canned | 2 |
| Green beans | 0 |
| Hummus | 10 |
| Kidney beans, red | 1 |
| Kidney beans,white | 1 |
| Lentils | 0 |
| Lima | 1 |

fat (grams)

\* Unless otherwise indicated, counts are based on 1/2 cup
tofu or cooked beans or one-ounce servings of raw nuts or
seeds.

## NUTS, BEANS AND SEEDS*: Part 2

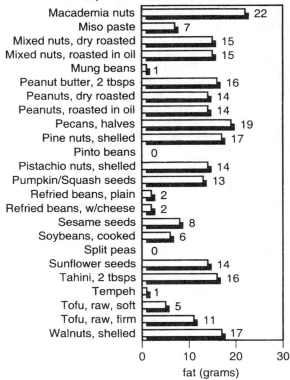

| | fat (grams) |
|---|---|
| Macademia nuts | 22 |
| Miso paste | 7 |
| Mixed nuts, dry roasted | 15 |
| Mixed nuts, roasted in oil | 15 |
| Mung beans | 1 |
| Peanut butter, 2 tbsps | 16 |
| Peanuts, dry roasted | 14 |
| Peanuts, roasted in oil | 14 |
| Pecans, halves | 19 |
| Pine nuts, shelled | 17 |
| Pinto beans | 0 |
| Pistachio nuts, shelled | 14 |
| Pumpkin/Squash seeds | 13 |
| Refried beans, plain | 2 |
| Refried beans, w/cheese | 2 |
| Sesame seeds | 8 |
| Soybeans, cooked | 6 |
| Split peas | 0 |
| Sunflower seeds | 14 |
| Tahini, 2 tbsps | 16 |
| Tempeh | 1 |
| Tofu, raw, soft | 5 |
| Tofu, raw, firm | 11 |
| Walnuts, shelled | 17 |

fat (grams)

\* Unless otherwise indicated, counts are based on 1/2 cup
tofu or cooked beans or one-ounce servings of raw nuts or
seeds.

**OILS AND FATS***

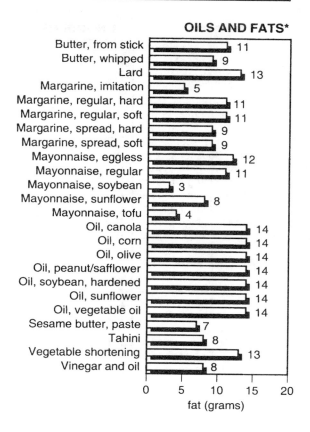

| | fat (grams) |
|---|---|
| Butter, from stick | 11 |
| Butter, whipped | 9 |
| Lard | 13 |
| Margarine, imitation | 5 |
| Margarine, regular, hard | 11 |
| Margarine, regular, soft | 11 |
| Margarine, spread, hard | 9 |
| Margarine, spread, soft | 9 |
| Mayonnaise, eggless | 12 |
| Mayonnaise, regular | 11 |
| Mayonnaise, soybean | 3 |
| Mayonnaise, sunflower | 8 |
| Mayonnaise, tofu | 4 |
| Oil, canola | 14 |
| Oil, corn | 14 |
| Oil, olive | 14 |
| Oil, peanut/safflower | 14 |
| Oil, soybean, hardened | 14 |
| Oil, sunflower | 14 |
| Oil, vegetable oil | 14 |
| Sesame butter, paste | 7 |
| Tahini | 8 |
| Vegetable shortening | 13 |
| Vinegar and oil | 8 |

* Counts are based on 1-tablespoon servings.

## PASTA, WHOLE GRAINS , RICE & NOODLES*, Part 1

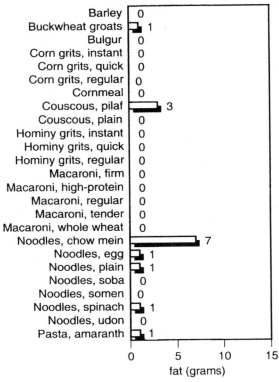

| | fat (grams) |
|---|---|
| Barley | 0 |
| Buckwheat groats | 1 |
| Bulgur | 0 |
| Corn grits, instant | 0 |
| Corn grits, quick | 0 |
| Corn grits, regular | 0 |
| Cornmeal | 0 |
| Couscous, pilaf | 3 |
| Couscous, plain | 0 |
| Hominy grits, instant | 0 |
| Hominy grits, quick | 0 |
| Hominy grits, regular | 0 |
| Macaroni, firm | 0 |
| Macaroni, high-protein | 0 |
| Macaroni, regular | 0 |
| Macaroni, tender | 0 |
| Macaroni, whole wheat | 0 |
| Noodles, chow mein | 7 |
| Noodles, egg | 1 |
| Noodles, plain | 1 |
| Noodles, soba | 0 |
| Noodles, somen | 0 |
| Noodles, spinach | 1 |
| Noodles, udon | 0 |
| Pasta, amaranth | 1 |

fat (grams)

* Counts are based on cooked, 1/2-cup servings.

52

### PASTA, WHOLE GRAINS , RICE & NOODLES*, Part 2

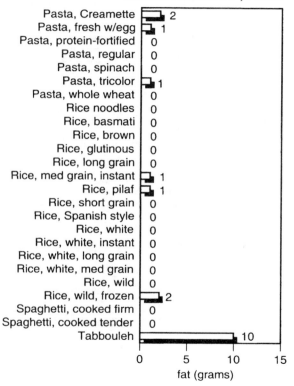

| | fat (grams) |
|---|---|
| Pasta, Creamette | 2 |
| Pasta, fresh w/egg | 1 |
| Pasta, protein-fortified | 0 |
| Pasta, regular | 0 |
| Pasta, spinach | 0 |
| Pasta, tricolor | 1 |
| Pasta, whole wheat | 0 |
| Rice noodles | 0 |
| Rice, basmati | 0 |
| Rice, brown | 0 |
| Rice, glutinous | 0 |
| Rice, long grain | 0 |
| Rice, med grain, instant | 1 |
| Rice, pilaf | 1 |
| Rice, short grain | 0 |
| Rice, Spanish style | 0 |
| Rice, white | 0 |
| Rice, white, instant | 0 |
| Rice, white, long grain | 0 |
| Rice, white, med grain | 0 |
| Rice, wild | 0 |
| Rice, wild, frozen | 2 |
| Spaghetti, cooked firm | 0 |
| Spaghetti, cooked tender | 0 |
| Tabbouleh | 10 |

* Counts are based on cooked, 1/2-cup servings.

53

## Poultry: CHICKEN, TURKEY, AND OTHER FOWL*

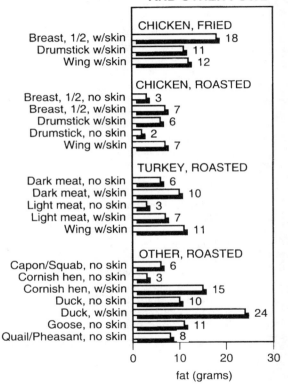

CHICKEN, FRIED
Breast, 1/2, w/skin — 18
Drumstick w/skin — 11
Wing w/skin — 12

CHICKEN, ROASTED
Breast, 1/2, no skin — 3
Breast, 1/2, w/skin — 7
Drumstick w/skin — 6
Drumstick, no skin — 2
Wing w/skin — 7

TURKEY, ROASTED
Dark meat, no skin — 6
Dark meat, w/skin — 10
Light meat, no skin — 3
Light meat, w/skin — 7
Wing w/skin — 11

OTHER, ROASTED
Capon/Squab, no skin — 6
Cornish hen, no skin — 3
Cornish hen, w/skin — 15
Duck, no skin — 10
Duck, w/skin — 24
Goose, no skin — 11
Quail/Pheasant, no skin — 8

0    10    20    30

fat (grams)

* Unless otherwise indicated, counts are based on 3-ounce servings.

## SALAD BAR CHOICES*

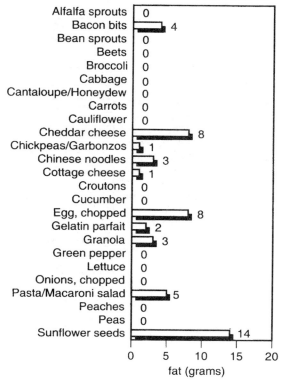

| Salad Bar Choice | fat (grams) |
|---|---|
| Alfalfa sprouts | 0 |
| Bacon bits | 4 |
| Bean sprouts | 0 |
| Beets | 0 |
| Broccoli | 0 |
| Cabbage | 0 |
| Cantaloupe/Honeydew | 0 |
| Carrots | 0 |
| Cauliflower | 0 |
| Cheddar cheese | 8 |
| Chickpeas/Garbonzos | 1 |
| Chinese noodles | 3 |
| Cottage cheese | 1 |
| Croutons | 0 |
| Cucumber | 0 |
| Egg, chopped | 8 |
| Gelatin parfait | 2 |
| Granola | 3 |
| Green pepper | 0 |
| Lettuce | 0 |
| Onions, chopped | 0 |
| Pasta/Macaroni salad | 5 |
| Peaches | 0 |
| Peas | 0 |
| Sunflower seeds | 14 |

fat (grams)

*Counts are based on one-quarter cup servings.

55

## SALAD DRESSING*

| Salad Dressing | fat (grams) |
|---|---|
| Blue cheese, low-cal | 2 |
| Blue cheese, reg | 6 |
| Caesar | 8 |
| Creamy Italian, low-cal | 2 |
| Creamy Italian, regular | 6 |
| French, low-cal | 2 |
| French, regular | 9 |
| Garlic, creamy | 8 |
| Garlic, regular | 5 |
| Honey mustard | 3 |
| Italian, low-cal | 0 |
| Italian, regular | 9 |
| Mayonnaise, light | 5 |
| Mayonnaise, low-fat | 1 |
| Mayonnaise, reg | 11 |
| Miracle Whip, light | 4 |
| Miracle Whip, regular | 7 |
| Oil & vinegar | 8 |
| Oil & vinegar dressing | 4 |
| Onion & chives | 7 |
| Ranch | 8 |
| Russian/Thous Island, low-cal | 1 |
| Russian/Thous Island, reg | 5 |
| Vinaigrette, low-cal | 3 |
| Vinaigrette, regular | 6 |

fat (grams) — 0 5 10 15

\* For ease of comparison, counts are based on single
tablespoon servings. Adjust counts to reflect quantities
consumed.

## SEAFOOD*, Part 1

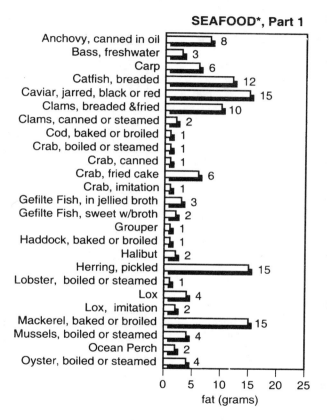

| Item | fat (grams) |
|------|-------------|
| Anchovy, canned in oil | 8 |
| Bass, freshwater | 3 |
| Carp | 6 |
| Catfish, breaded | 12 |
| Caviar, jarred, black or red | 15 |
| Clams, breaded &fried | 10 |
| Clams, canned or steamed | 2 |
| Cod, baked or broiled | 1 |
| Crab, boiled or steamed | 1 |
| Crab, canned | 1 |
| Crab, fried cake | 6 |
| Crab, imitation | 1 |
| Gefilte Fish, in jellied broth | 3 |
| Gefilte Fish, sweet w/broth | 2 |
| Grouper | 1 |
| Haddock, baked or broiled | 1 |
| Halibut | 2 |
| Herring, pickled | 15 |
| Lobster, boiled or steamed | 1 |
| Lox | 4 |
| Lox, imitation | 2 |
| Mackerel, baked or broiled | 15 |
| Mussels, boiled or steamed | 4 |
| Ocean Perch | 2 |
| Oyster, boiled or steamed | 4 |

fat (grams) — scale: 0  5  10  15  20  25

* Counts are based on 3-ounce servings. Canned seafood items are assumed to be drained.

Alphabetical Chart
(for Hi-Low Comparison Charts, see pages 83 - 164)

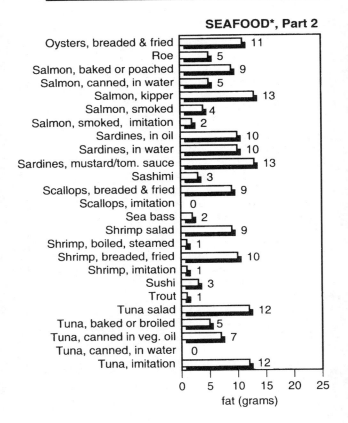

**SEAFOOD\*, Part 2**

| Item | fat (grams) |
|------|-------------|
| Oysters, breaded & fried | 11 |
| Roe | 5 |
| Salmon, baked or poached | 9 |
| Salmon, canned, in water | 5 |
| Salmon, kipper | 13 |
| Salmon, smoked | 4 |
| Salmon, smoked, imitation | 2 |
| Sardines, in oil | 10 |
| Sardines, in water | 10 |
| Sardines, mustard/tom. sauce | 13 |
| Sashimi | 3 |
| Scallops, breaded & fried | 9 |
| Scallops, imitation | 0 |
| Sea bass | 2 |
| Shrimp salad | 9 |
| Shrimp, boiled, steamed | 1 |
| Shrimp, breaded, fried | 10 |
| Shrimp, imitation | 1 |
| Sushi | 3 |
| Trout | 1 |
| Tuna salad | 12 |
| Tuna, baked or broiled | 5 |
| Tuna, canned in veg. oil | 7 |
| Tuna, canned, in water | 0 |
| Tuna, imitation | 12 |

fat (grams) — 0 5 10 15 20 25

\* Counts are based on 3-ounce servings. Canned seafood
items are assumed to be drained.

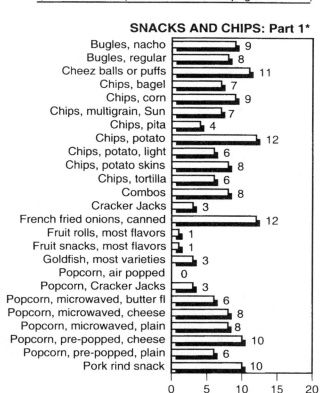

## SNACKS AND CHIPS: Part 1*

| Food | fat (grams) |
|---|---|
| Bugles, nacho | 9 |
| Bugles, regular | 8 |
| Cheez balls or puffs | 11 |
| Chips, bagel | 7 |
| Chips, corn | 9 |
| Chips, multigrain, Sun | 7 |
| Chips, pita | 4 |
| Chips, potato | 12 |
| Chips, potato, light | 6 |
| Chips, potato skins | 8 |
| Chips, tortilla | 6 |
| Combos | 8 |
| Cracker Jacks | 3 |
| French fried onions, canned | 12 |
| Fruit rolls, most flavors | 1 |
| Fruit snacks, most flavors | 1 |
| Goldfish, most varieties | 3 |
| Popcorn, air popped | 0 |
| Popcorn, Cracker Jacks | 3 |
| Popcorn, microwaved, butter fl | 6 |
| Popcorn, microwaved, cheese | 8 |
| Popcorn, microwaved, plain | 8 |
| Popcorn, pre-popped, cheese | 10 |
| Popcorn, pre-popped, plain | 6 |
| Pork rind snack | 10 |

fat (grams)

\* For ease of comparison, counts are based on one-ounce
servings. For popcorn, 1 ounce unpopped = 2 cups popped.
Adjust count to reflect amount consumed.

### SNACKS AND CHIPS: Part 2*

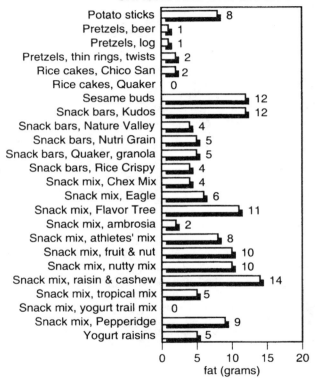

| | fat (grams) |
|---|---|
| Potato sticks | 8 |
| Pretzels, beer | 1 |
| Pretzels, log | 1 |
| Pretzels, thin rings, twists | 2 |
| Rice cakes, Chico San | 2 |
| Rice cakes, Quaker | 0 |
| Sesame buds | 12 |
| Snack bars, Kudos | 12 |
| Snack bars, Nature Valley | 4 |
| Snack bars, Nutri Grain | 5 |
| Snack bars, Quaker, granola | 5 |
| Snack bars, Rice Crispy | 4 |
| Snack mix, Chex Mix | 4 |
| Snack mix, Eagle | 6 |
| Snack mix, Flavor Tree | 11 |
| Snack mix, ambrosia | 2 |
| Snack mix, athletes' mix | 8 |
| Snack mix, fruit & nut | 10 |
| Snack mix, nutty mix | 10 |
| Snack mix, raisin & cashew | 14 |
| Snack mix, tropical mix | 5 |
| Snack mix, yogurt trail mix | 0 |
| Snack mix, Pepperidge | 9 |
| Yogurt raisins | 5 |

\* For ease of comparison, counts are based on one-ounce
servings. For popcorn, 1 ounce unpopped = 2 cups popped.
Adjust count to reflect amount consumed.

## SOUP*: Part 1

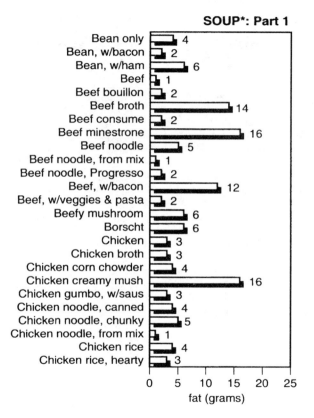

| | fat (grams) |
|---|---|
| Bean only | 4 |
| Bean, w/bacon | 2 |
| Bean, w/ham | 6 |
| Beef | 1 |
| Beef bouillon | 2 |
| Beef broth | 14 |
| Beef consume | 2 |
| Beef minestrone | 16 |
| Beef noodle | 5 |
| Beef noodle, from mix | 1 |
| Beef noodle, Progresso | 2 |
| Beef, w/bacon | 12 |
| Beef, w/veggies & pasta | 2 |
| Beefy mushroom | 6 |
| Borscht | 6 |
| Chicken | 3 |
| Chicken broth | 3 |
| Chicken corn chowder | 4 |
| Chicken creamy mush | 16 |
| Chicken gumbo, w/saus | 3 |
| Chicken noodle, canned | 4 |
| Chicken noodle, chunky | 5 |
| Chicken noodle, from mix | 1 |
| Chicken rice | 4 |
| Chicken rice, hearty | 3 |

fat (grams) — axis: 0  5  10  15  20  25

\* Unless otherwise indicated, counts are based on one-cup servings.

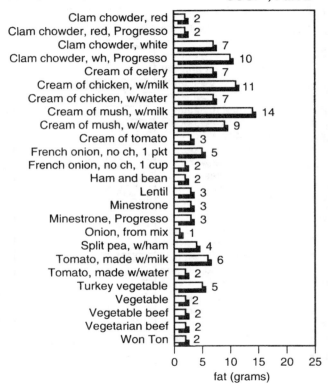

# Alphabetical Chart
(for Hi-Low Comparison Charts, see pages 83 - 164)

## SOUP*, Part 2

| Food | fat (grams) |
|------|-------------|
| Clam chowder, red | 2 |
| Clam chowder, red, Progresso | 2 |
| Clam chowder, white | 7 |
| Clam chowder, wh, Progresso | 10 |
| Cream of celery | 7 |
| Cream of chicken, w/milk | 11 |
| Cream of chicken, w/water | 7 |
| Cream of mush, w/milk | 14 |
| Cream of mush, w/water | 9 |
| Cream of tomato | 3 |
| French onion, no ch, 1 pkt | 5 |
| French onion, no ch, 1 cup | 2 |
| Ham and bean | 2 |
| Lentil | 3 |
| Minestrone | 3 |
| Minestrone, Progresso | 3 |
| Onion, from mix | 1 |
| Split pea, w/ham | 4 |
| Tomato, made w/milk | 6 |
| Tomato, made w/water | 2 |
| Turkey vegetable | 5 |
| Vegetable | 2 |
| Vegetable beef | 2 |
| Vegetarian beef | 2 |
| Won Ton | 2 |

* Unless otherwise indicated, counts are based on one-cup servings.

## Sweets: CAKES*, Part 1

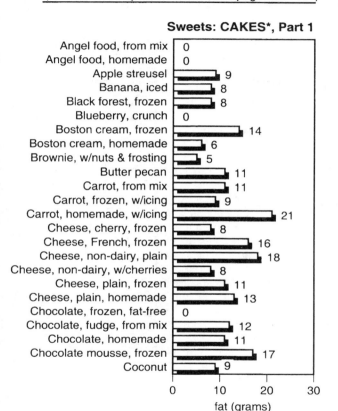

| Food | fat (grams) |
|------|-------------|
| Angel food, from mix | 0 |
| Angel food, homemade | 0 |
| Apple streusel | 9 |
| Banana, iced | 8 |
| Black forest, frozen | 8 |
| Blueberry, crunch | 0 |
| Boston cream, frozen | 14 |
| Boston cream, homemade | 6 |
| Brownie, w/nuts & frosting | 5 |
| Butter pecan | 11 |
| Carrot, from mix | 11 |
| Carrot, frozen, w/icing | 9 |
| Carrot, homemade, w/icing | 21 |
| Cheese, cherry, frozen | 8 |
| Cheese, French, frozen | 16 |
| Cheese, non-dairy, plain | 18 |
| Cheese, non-dairy, w/cherries | 8 |
| Cheese, plain, frozen | 11 |
| Cheese, plain, homemade | 13 |
| Chocolate, frozen, fat-free | 0 |
| Chocolate, fudge, from mix | 12 |
| Chocolate, homemade | 11 |
| Chocolate mousse, frozen | 17 |
| Coconut | 9 |

fat (grams)

* Counts are based on average-size pieces and slices,
  where appropriate, as indicated on package.

## Sweets: CAKES*, Part 2

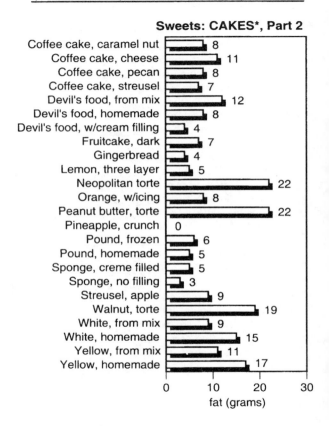

| | fat (grams) |
|---|---|
| Coffee cake, caramel nut | 8 |
| Coffee cake, cheese | 11 |
| Coffee cake, pecan | 8 |
| Coffee cake, streusel | 7 |
| Devil's food, from mix | 12 |
| Devil's food, homemade | 8 |
| Devil's food, w/cream filling | 4 |
| Fruitcake, dark | 7 |
| Gingerbread | 4 |
| Lemon, three layer | 5 |
| Neopolitan torte | 22 |
| Orange, w/icing | 8 |
| Peanut butter, torte | 22 |
| Pineapple, crunch | 0 |
| Pound, frozen | 6 |
| Pound, homemade | 5 |
| Sponge, creme filled | 5 |
| Sponge, no filling | 3 |
| Streusel, apple | 9 |
| Walnut, torte | 19 |
| White, from mix | 9 |
| White, homemade | 15 |
| Yellow, from mix | 11 |
| Yellow, homemade | 17 |

* Counts are based on average-size pieces and slices,
  where appropriate, as indicated on package.

## Sweets: SNACK CAKES*

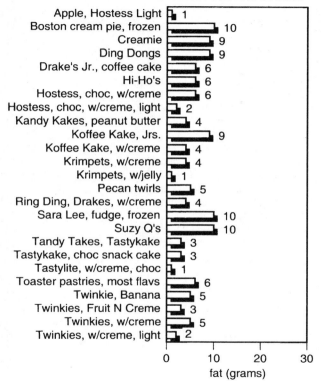

| | fat (grams) |
|---|---|
| Apple, Hostess Light | 1 |
| Boston cream pie, frozen | 10 |
| Creamie | 9 |
| Ding Dongs | 9 |
| Drake's Jr., coffee cake | 6 |
| Hi-Ho's | 6 |
| Hostess, choc, w/creme | 6 |
| Hostess, choc, w/creme, light | 2 |
| Kandy Kakes, peanut butter | 4 |
| Koffee Kake, Jrs. | 9 |
| Koffee Kake, w/creme | 4 |
| Krimpets, w/creme | 4 |
| Krimpets, w/jelly | 1 |
| Pecan twirls | 5 |
| Ring Ding, Drakes, w/creme | 4 |
| Sara Lee, fudge, frozen | 10 |
| Suzy Q's | 10 |
| Tandy Takes, Tastykake | 3 |
| Tastykake, choc snack cake | 3 |
| Tastylite, w/creme, choc | 1 |
| Toaster pastries, most flavs | 6 |
| Twinkie, Banana | 5 |
| Twinkies, Fruit N Creme | 3 |
| Twinkies, w/creme | 5 |
| Twinkies, w/creme, light | 2 |

0    10    20    30
fat (grams)

\* Counts are based on average-size pieces and slices,
  where appropriate, as indicated on package.

**Sweets: CANDY\*, Part 1**

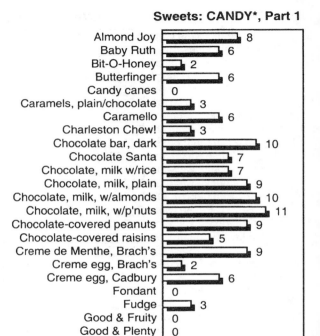

| | fat (grams) |
|---|---|
| Almond Joy | 8 |
| Baby Ruth | 6 |
| Bit-O-Honey | 2 |
| Butterfinger | 6 |
| Candy canes | 0 |
| Caramels, plain/chocolate | 3 |
| Caramello | 6 |
| Charleston Chew! | 3 |
| Chocolate bar, dark | 10 |
| Chocolate Santa | 7 |
| Chocolate, milk w/rice | 7 |
| Chocolate, milk, plain | 9 |
| Chocolate, milk, w/almonds | 10 |
| Chocolate, milk, w/p'nuts | 11 |
| Chocolate-covered peanuts | 9 |
| Chocolate-covered raisins | 5 |
| Creme de Menthe, Brach's | 9 |
| Creme egg, Brach's | 2 |
| Creme egg, Cadbury | 6 |
| Fondant | 0 |
| Fudge | 3 |
| Good & Fruity | 0 |
| Good & Plenty | 0 |
| Gum drops | 0 |
| Gummy Bears | 0 |

\* For ease of comparison, counts are based on one-ounce servings. Adjust counts to reflect quantities consumed.

### Sweets: CANDY\*, Part 2

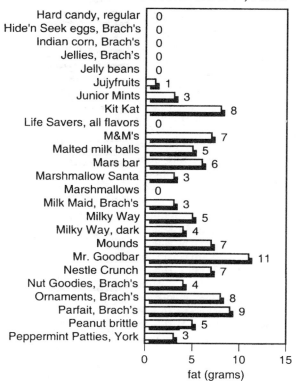

| | fat (grams) |
|---|---|
| Hard candy, regular | 0 |
| Hide'n Seek eggs, Brach's | 0 |
| Indian corn, Brach's | 0 |
| Jellies, Brach's | 0 |
| Jelly beans | 0 |
| Jujyfruits | 1 |
| Junior Mints | 3 |
| Kit Kat | 8 |
| Life Savers, all flavors | 0 |
| M&M's | 7 |
| Malted milk balls | 5 |
| Mars bar | 6 |
| Marshmallow Santa | 3 |
| Marshmallows | 0 |
| Milk Maid, Brach's | 3 |
| Milky Way | 5 |
| Milky Way, dark | 4 |
| Mounds | 7 |
| Mr. Goodbar | 11 |
| Nestle Crunch | 7 |
| Nut Goodies, Brach's | 4 |
| Ornaments, Brach's | 8 |
| Parfait, Brach's | 9 |
| Peanut brittle | 5 |
| Peppermint Patties, York | 3 |

\* For ease of comparison, counts are based on one-ounce servings. Adjust counts to reflect quantities consumed.

## Sweets: CANDY*, Part 3

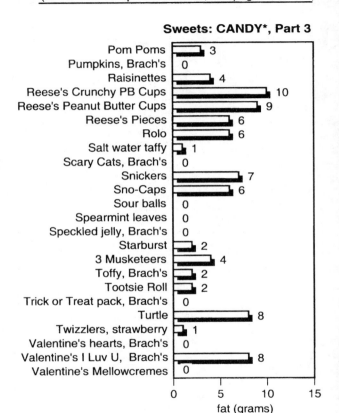

fat (grams)

* For ease of comparison, counts are based on one-ounce
servings. Adjust counts to reflect quantities consumed.

### Sweets: COOKIES*, Part 1

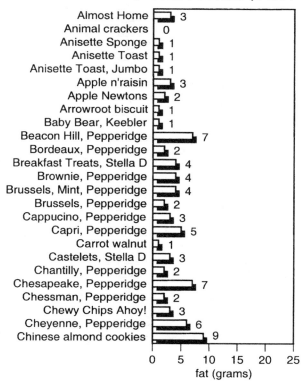

| Cookie | fat (grams) |
|---|---|
| Almost Home | 3 |
| Animal crackers | 0 |
| Anisette Sponge | 1 |
| Anisette Toast | 1 |
| Anisette Toast, Jumbo | 1 |
| Apple n'raisin | 3 |
| Apple Newtons | 2 |
| Arrowroot biscuit | 1 |
| Baby Bear, Keebler | 1 |
| Beacon Hill, Pepperidge | 7 |
| Bordeaux, Pepperidge | 2 |
| Breakfast Treats, Stella D | 4 |
| Brownie, Pepperidge | 4 |
| Brussels, Mint, Pepperidge | 4 |
| Brussels, Pepperidge | 2 |
| Cappucino, Pepperidge | 3 |
| Capri, Pepperidge | 5 |
| Carrot walnut | 1 |
| Castelets, Stella D | 3 |
| Chantilly, Pepperidge | 2 |
| Chesapeake, Pepperidge | 7 |
| Chessman, Pepperidge | 2 |
| Chewy Chips Ahoy! | 3 |
| Cheyenne, Pepperidge | 6 |
| Chinese almond cookies | 9 |

fat (grams)

* NOTE: For ease of comparison, counts are based on
single cookie servings. When more than one cookie is
consumed, counts should be adjusted accordingly.

## Sweets: COOKIES, Part 2

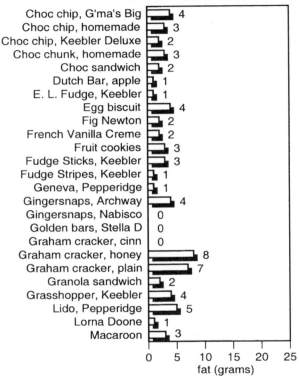

| Cookie | fat (grams) |
|---|---|
| Choc chip, G'ma's Big | 4 |
| Choc chip, homemade | 3 |
| Choc chip, Keebler Deluxe | 2 |
| Choc chunk, homemade | 3 |
| Choc sandwich | 2 |
| Dutch Bar, apple | 1 |
| E. L. Fudge, Keebler | 1 |
| Egg biscuit | 4 |
| Fig Newton | 2 |
| French Vanilla Creme | 2 |
| Fruit cookies | 3 |
| Fudge Sticks, Keebler | 3 |
| Fudge Stripes, Keebler | 1 |
| Geneva, Pepperidge | 1 |
| Gingersnaps, Archway | 4 |
| Gingersnaps, Nabisco | 0 |
| Golden bars, Stella D | 0 |
| Graham cracker, cinn | 0 |
| Graham cracker, honey | 8 |
| Graham cracker, plain | 7 |
| Granola sandwich | 2 |
| Grasshopper, Keebler | 4 |
| Lido, Pepperidge | 5 |
| Lorna Doone | 1 |
| Macaroon | 3 |

fat (grams)  0  5  10  15  20  25

\* NOTE: For ease of comparison, counts are based on
single cookie servings. When more than one cookie is
consumed, counts should be adjusted accordingly.

70

## Sweets: COOKIES*, Part 3

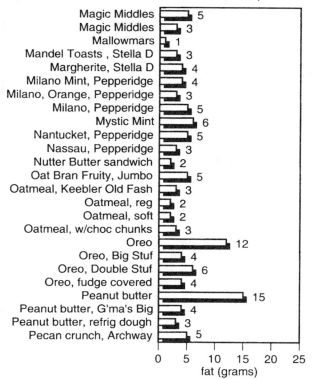

| Cookie | fat (grams) |
|---|---|
| Magic Middles | 5 |
| Magic Middles | 3 |
| Mallowmars | 1 |
| Mandel Toasts , Stella D | 3 |
| Margherite, Stella D | 4 |
| Milano Mint, Pepperidge | 4 |
| Milano, Orange, Pepperidge | 3 |
| Milano, Pepperidge | 5 |
| Mystic Mint | 6 |
| Nantucket, Pepperidge | 5 |
| Nassau, Pepperidge | 3 |
| Nutter Butter sandwich | 2 |
| Oat Bran Fruity, Jumbo | 5 |
| Oatmeal, Keebler Old Fash | 3 |
| Oatmeal, reg | 2 |
| Oatmeal, soft | 2 |
| Oatmeal, w/choc chunks | 3 |
| Oreo | 12 |
| Oreo, Big Stuf | 4 |
| Oreo, Double Stuf | 6 |
| Oreo, fudge covered | 4 |
| Peanut butter | 15 |
| Peanut butter, G'ma's Big | 4 |
| Peanut butter, refrig dough | 3 |
| Pecan crunch, Archway | 5 |

fat (grams): 0  5  10  15  20  25

* NOTE: For ease of comparison, counts are based on
single cookie servings. When more than one cookie is
consumed, counts should be adjusted accordingly.

### Sweets: COOKIES*, Part 4

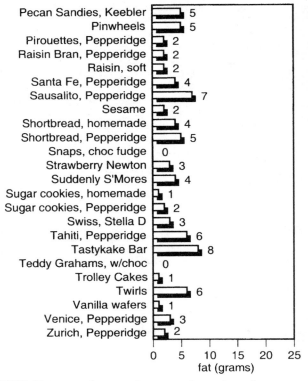

| | fat (grams) |
|---|---|
| Pecan Sandies, Keebler | 5 |
| Pinwheels | 5 |
| Pirouettes, Pepperidge | 2 |
| Raisin Bran, Pepperidge | 2 |
| Raisin, soft | 2 |
| Santa Fe, Pepperidge | 4 |
| Sausalito, Pepperidge | 7 |
| Sesame | 2 |
| Shortbread, homemade | 4 |
| Shortbread, Pepperidge | 5 |
| Snaps, choc fudge | 0 |
| Strawberry Newton | 3 |
| Suddenly S'Mores | 4 |
| Sugar cookies, homemade | 1 |
| Sugar cookies, Pepperidge | 2 |
| Swiss, Stella D | 3 |
| Tahiti, Pepperidge | 6 |
| Tastykake Bar | 8 |
| Teddy Grahams, w/choc | 0 |
| Trolley Cakes | 1 |
| Twirls | 6 |
| Vanilla wafers | 1 |
| Venice, Pepperidge | 3 |
| Zurich, Pepperidge | 2 |

0   5   10   15   20   25
fat (grams)

\* NOTE: For ease of comparison, counts are based on
single cookie servings. When more than one cookie is
consumed, counts should be adjusted accordingly.

72

**Sweets: DONUTS\***

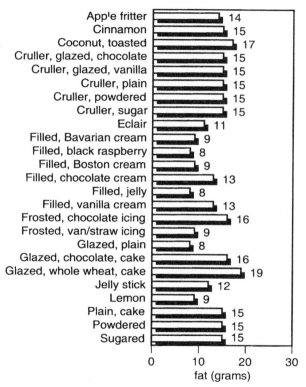

| Donut | fat (grams) |
|---|---|
| Apple fritter | 14 |
| Cinnamon | 15 |
| Coconut, toasted | 17 |
| Cruller, glazed, chocolate | 15 |
| Cruller, glazed, vanilla | 15 |
| Cruller, plain | 15 |
| Cruller, powdered | 15 |
| Cruller, sugar | 15 |
| Eclair | 11 |
| Filled, Bavarian cream | 9 |
| Filled, black raspberry | 8 |
| Filled, Boston cream | 9 |
| Filled, chocolate cream | 13 |
| Filled, jelly | 8 |
| Filled, vanilla cream | 13 |
| Frosted, chocolate icing | 16 |
| Frosted, van/straw icing | 9 |
| Glazed, plain | 8 |
| Glazed, chocolate, cake | 16 |
| Glazed, whole wheat, cake | 19 |
| Jelly stick | 12 |
| Lemon | 9 |
| Plain, cake | 15 |
| Powdered | 15 |
| Sugared | 15 |

fat (grams)

\* Counts are based on average-size donuts.

**Sweets: GUM & MINTS***

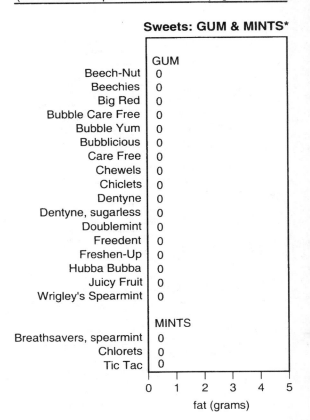

| | fat (grams) |
|---|---|
| **GUM** | |
| Beech-Nut | 0 |
| Beechies | 0 |
| Big Red | 0 |
| Bubble Care Free | 0 |
| Bubble Yum | 0 |
| Bubblicious | 0 |
| Care Free | 0 |
| Chewels | 0 |
| Chiclets | 0 |
| Dentyne | 0 |
| Dentyne, sugarless | 0 |
| Doublemint | 0 |
| Freedent | 0 |
| Freshen-Up | 0 |
| Hubba Bubba | 0 |
| Juicy Fruit | 0 |
| Wrigley's Spearmint | 0 |
| **MINTS** | |
| Breathsavers, spearmint | 0 |
| Chlorets | 0 |
| Tic Tac | 0 |

\* Counts are based on single sticks or mints.

**Sweets: ICE CREAM***

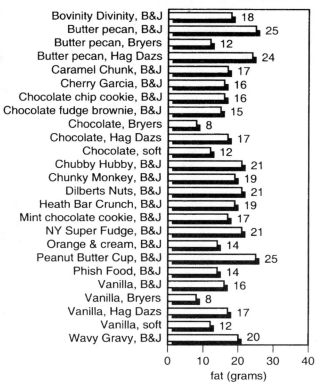

| Ice Cream | fat (grams) |
|---|---|
| Bovinity Divinity, B&J | 18 |
| Butter pecan, B&J | 25 |
| Butter pecan, Bryers | 12 |
| Butter pecan, Hag Dazs | 24 |
| Caramel Chunk, B&J | 17 |
| Cherry Garcia, B&J | 16 |
| Chocolate chip cookie, B&J | 16 |
| Chocolate fudge brownie, B&J | 15 |
| Chocolate, Bryers | 8 |
| Chocolate, Hag Dazs | 17 |
| Chocolate, soft | 12 |
| Chubby Hubby, B&J | 21 |
| Chunky Monkey, B&J | 19 |
| Dilberts Nuts, B&J | 21 |
| Heath Bar Crunch, B&J | 19 |
| Mint chocolate cookie, B&J | 17 |
| NY Super Fudge, B&J | 21 |
| Orange & cream, B&J | 14 |
| Peanut Butter Cup, B&J | 25 |
| Phish Food, B&J | 14 |
| Vanilla, B&J | 16 |
| Vanilla, Bryers | 8 |
| Vanilla, Hag Dazs | 17 |
| Vanilla, soft | 12 |
| Wavy Gravy, B&J | 20 |

fat (grams)

* Counts are based on one-half cup servings. "B&J"
designates Ben & Jerry's brand.

## Sweets: ICE CREAM CONES & BARS, ICE CREAM ALTERNATIVES AND PUDDINGS*

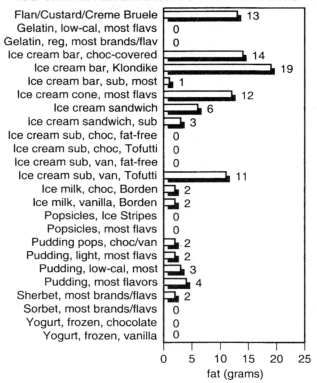

| | fat (grams) |
|---|---|
| Flan/Custard/Creme Bruele | 13 |
| Gelatin, low-cal, most flavs | 0 |
| Gelatin, reg, most brands/flav | 0 |
| Ice cream bar, choc-covered | 14 |
| Ice cream bar, Klondike | 19 |
| Ice cream bar, sub, most | 1 |
| Ice cream cone, most flavs | 12 |
| Ice cream sandwich | 6 |
| Ice cream sandwich, sub | 3 |
| Ice cream sub, choc, fat-free | 0 |
| Ice cream sub, choc, Tofutti | 0 |
| Ice cream sub, van, fat-free | 0 |
| Ice cream sub, van, Tofutti | 11 |
| Ice milk, choc, Borden | 2 |
| Ice milk, vanilla, Borden | 2 |
| Popsicles, Ice Stripes | 0 |
| Popsicles, most flavs | 0 |
| Pudding pops, choc/van | 2 |
| Pudding, light, most flavs | 2 |
| Pudding, low-cal, most | 3 |
| Pudding, most flavors | 4 |
| Sherbet, most brands/flavs | 2 |
| Sorbet, most brands/flavs | 0 |
| Yogurt, frozen, chocolate | 0 |
| Yogurt, frozen, vanilla | 0 |

0    5    10    15    20    25
fat (grams)

\* Counts are based on average- or one-half cup servings.
"Sub" designates non-dairy, ice cream substitute.

## Sweets: PIES*

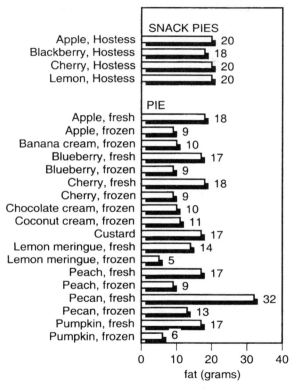

SNACK PIES
Apple, Hostess — 20
Blackberry, Hostess — 18
Cherry, Hostess — 20
Lemon, Hostess — 20

PIE
Apple, fresh — 18
Apple, frozen — 9
Banana cream, frozen — 10
Blueberry, fresh — 17
Blueberry, frozen — 9
Cherry, fresh — 18
Cherry, frozen — 9
Chocolate cream, frozen — 10
Coconut cream, frozen — 11
Custard — 17
Lemon meringue, fresh — 14
Lemon meringue, frozen — 5
Peach, fresh — 17
Peach, frozen — 9
Pecan, fresh — 32
Pecan, frozen — 13
Pumpkin, fresh — 17
Pumpkin, frozen — 6

fat (grams)
0    10    20    30    40

\* Counts are based on average-size pieces and slices,
  where appropriate, as indicated on package.

## Sweets: SUGARS, SYRUPS, TOPPINGS AND JAMS*

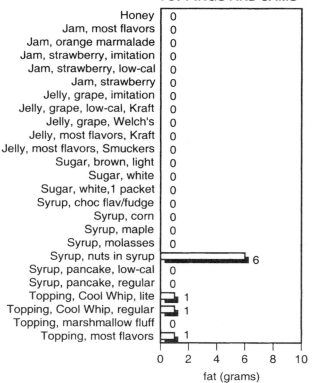

| | fat (grams) |
|---|---|
| Honey | 0 |
| Jam, most flavors | 0 |
| Jam, orange marmalade | 0 |
| Jam, strawberry, imitation | 0 |
| Jam, strawberry, low-cal | 0 |
| Jam, strawberry | 0 |
| Jelly, grape, imitation | 0 |
| Jelly, grape, low-cal, Kraft | 0 |
| Jelly, grape, Welch's | 0 |
| Jelly, most flavors, Kraft | 0 |
| Jelly, most flavors, Smuckers | 0 |
| Sugar, brown, light | 0 |
| Sugar, white | 0 |
| Sugar, white, 1 packet | 0 |
| Syrup, choc flav/fudge | 0 |
| Syrup, corn | 0 |
| Syrup, maple | 0 |
| Syrup, molasses | 0 |
| Syrup, nuts in syrup | 6 |
| Syrup, pancake, low-cal | 0 |
| Syrup, pancake, regular | 0 |
| Topping, Cool Whip, lite | 1 |
| Topping, Cool Whip, regular | 1 |
| Topping, marshmallow fluff | 0 |
| Topping, most flavors | 1 |

* Counts are based on single-tablespoon servings. Jams
and preserves can be assumed to have equal values.

## VEGETABLES*, Part 1

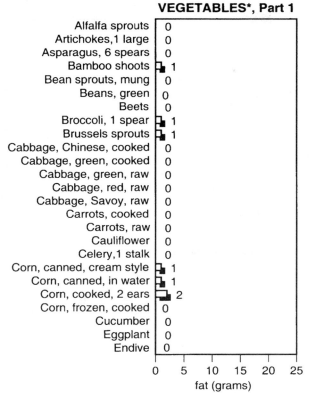

| | fat (grams) |
|---|---|
| Alfalfa sprouts | 0 |
| Artichokes, 1 large | 0 |
| Asparagus, 6 spears | 0 |
| Bamboo shoots | 1 |
| Bean sprouts, mung | 0 |
| Beans, green | 0 |
| Beets | 0 |
| Broccoli, 1 spear | 1 |
| Brussels sprouts | 1 |
| Cabbage, Chinese, cooked | 0 |
| Cabbage, green, cooked | 0 |
| Cabbage, green, raw | 0 |
| Cabbage, red, raw | 0 |
| Cabbage, Savoy, raw | 0 |
| Carrots, cooked | 0 |
| Carrots, raw | 0 |
| Cauliflower | 0 |
| Celery, 1 stalk | 0 |
| Corn, canned, cream style | 1 |
| Corn, canned, in water | 1 |
| Corn, cooked, 2 ears | 2 |
| Corn, frozen, cooked | 0 |
| Cucumber | 0 |
| Eggplant | 0 |
| Endive | 0 |

fat (grams) — 0   5   10   15   20   25

* Unless otherwise indicated, counts are based on one-cup
servings. For vegetable juices, see the Fruits & Juices
section.

**VEGETABLES\*, Part 2**

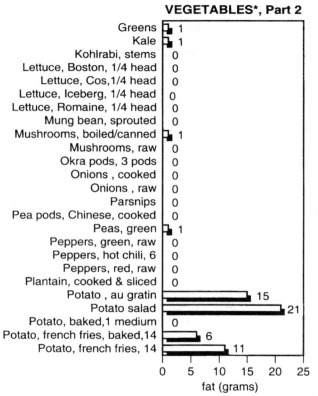

| | fat (grams) |
|---|---|
| Greens | 1 |
| Kale | 1 |
| Kohlrabi, stems | 0 |
| Lettuce, Boston, 1/4 head | 0 |
| Lettuce, Cos,1/4 head | 0 |
| Lettuce, Iceberg, 1/4 head | 0 |
| Lettuce, Romaine, 1/4 head | 0 |
| Mung bean, sprouted | 0 |
| Mushrooms, boiled/canned | 1 |
| Mushrooms, raw | 0 |
| Okra pods, 3 pods | 0 |
| Onions , cooked | 0 |
| Onions , raw | 0 |
| Parsnips | 0 |
| Pea pods, Chinese, cooked | 0 |
| Peas, green | 1 |
| Peppers, green, raw | 0 |
| Peppers, hot chili, 6 | 0 |
| Peppers, red, raw | 0 |
| Plantain, cooked & sliced | 0 |
| Potato , au gratin | 15 |
| Potato salad | 21 |
| Potato, baked,1 medium | 0 |
| Potato, french fries, baked,14 | 6 |
| Potato, french fries, 14 | 11 |

fat (grams)

\* Unless otherwise indicated, counts are based on one-cup
servings. For vegetable juices, see the Fruits & Juices
section.

## VEGETABLES*, Part 3

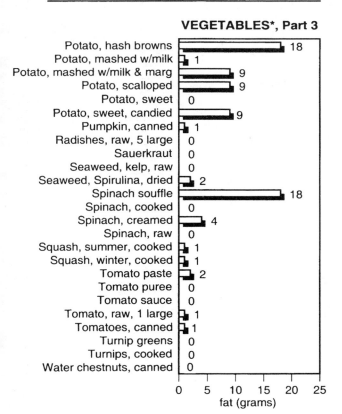

| | fat (grams) |
|---|---|
| Potato, hash browns | 18 |
| Potato, mashed w/milk | 1 |
| Potato, mashed w/milk & marg | 9 |
| Potato, scalloped | 9 |
| Potato, sweet | 0 |
| Potato, sweet, candied | 9 |
| Pumpkin, canned | 1 |
| Radishes, raw, 5 large | 0 |
| Sauerkraut | 0 |
| Seaweed, kelp, raw | 0 |
| Seaweed, Spirulina, dried | 2 |
| Spinach souffle | 18 |
| Spinach, cooked | 0 |
| Spinach, creamed | 4 |
| Spinach, raw | 0 |
| Squash, summer, cooked | 1 |
| Squash, winter, cooked | 1 |
| Tomato paste | 2 |
| Tomato puree | 0 |
| Tomato sauce | 0 |
| Tomato, raw, 1 large | 1 |
| Tomatoes, canned | 1 |
| Turnip greens | 0 |
| Turnips, cooked | 0 |
| Water chestnuts, canned | 0 |

\* Unless otherwise indicated, counts are based on one-cup servings. For vegetable juices, see the Fruits & Juices section.

## VEGETARIAN CHOICES*

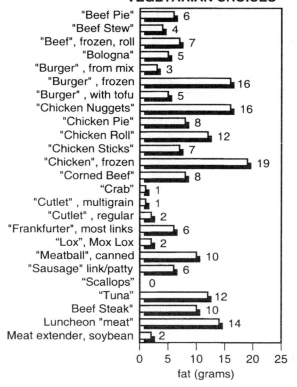

| Item | fat (grams) |
|------|-------------|
| "Beef Pie" | 6 |
| "Beef Stew" | 4 |
| "Beef", frozen, roll | 7 |
| "Bologna" | 5 |
| "Burger", from mix | 3 |
| "Burger", frozen | 16 |
| "Burger", with tofu | 5 |
| "Chicken Nuggets" | 16 |
| "Chicken Pie" | 8 |
| "Chicken Roll" | 12 |
| "Chicken Sticks" | 7 |
| "Chicken", frozen | 19 |
| "Corned Beef" | 8 |
| "Crab" | 1 |
| "Cutlet", multigrain | 1 |
| "Cutlet", regular | 2 |
| "Frankfurter", most links | 6 |
| "Lox", Mox Lox | 2 |
| "Meatball", canned | 10 |
| "Sausage" link/patty | 6 |
| "Scallops" | 0 |
| "Tuna" | 12 |
| Beef Steak" | 10 |
| Luncheon "meat" | 14 |
| Meat extender, soybean | 2 |

fat (grams)

\* Made from tofu, textured vegetable protein or a combination of both. Counts are based on 3-ounce servings.

# HI-LOW COMPARISON CHARTS

## BEVERAGES*, Part 1

| | fat (grams) |
|---|---|
| Amaretto | 0 |
| Apple juice | 0 |
| Apricot cordial | 0 |
| Apricot nectar | 0 |
| Beer, dark | 0 |
| Beer, light | 0 |
| Beer, regular | 0 |
| Carrot juice | 0 |
| Champagne | 0 |
| Clam & tomato cocktail | 0 |
| Club soda | 0 |
| Coffee | 0 |
| Coffee-flavor grain bev | 0 |
| Cola, regular | 0 |
| Cola, sugar-free | 0 |
| Cranberry juice cocktail | 0 |
| Cranberry juice, sweetened | 0 |
| Creme de Cacao | 0 |
| Creme de Menthe | 0 |
| Crystal Light, most flavors | 0 |
| Fruit punch drink | 0 |
| Gin | 0 |
| Ginger ale, regular | 0 |
| Ginger ale, sugar-free | 0 |
| Grape drink | 0 |

0   5   10   15   20   25
fat (grams)

* Counts for non-alcoholic drinks and beer are based on
8-fluid-ounce servings,  for wine on 3 1/2-fluid-ounce
servings and,  for hard liquor, on 1 1/2-fluid-ounce servings.

## BEVERAGES*, Part 2

| | fat (grams) |
|---|---|
| Grape juice | 0 |
| Grape soda | 0 |
| Grapefruit juice | 0 |
| Lemon-lime soda | 0 |
| Lemonade, from conc. | 0 |
| Limeade | 0 |
| Milk, nonfat | 0 |
| Milk, skim | 0 |
| Pineapple juice, unsweetened | 0 |
| Pineapple-grapefruit juice | 0 |
| Root beer, regular | 0 |
| Root beer, sugar-free | 0 |
| Rum | 0 |
| 7 Up, regular | 0 |
| 7 Up, sugar-free | 0 |
| Sprite, regular | 0 |
| Sprite, sugar-free | 0 |
| Tea | 0 |
| Tomato juice, 8 fl oz | 0 |
| Tonic water, regular | 0 |
| Tonic water, sugar-free | 0 |
| Vegetable juice cocktail | 0 |
| Vegetable juice, V-8 | 0 |
| Vodka | 0 |
| Whisky | 0 |

```
0    5    10   15   20   25
           fat (grams)
```

* Counts for non-alcoholic drinks and beer are based on
  8-fluid-ounce servings,  for wine on 3 1/2-fluid-ounce
  servings and,  for hard liquor, on 1 1/2-fluid-ounce servings.

## BEVERAGES*, Part 3

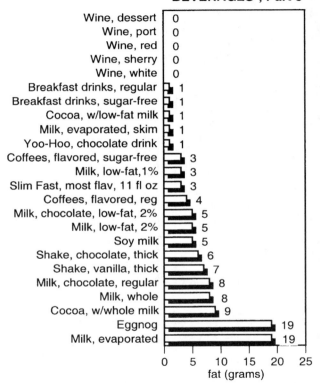

| | fat (grams) |
|---|---|
| Wine, dessert | 0 |
| Wine, port | 0 |
| Wine, red | 0 |
| Wine, sherry | 0 |
| Wine, white | 0 |
| Breakfast drinks, regular | 1 |
| Breakfast drinks, sugar-free | 1 |
| Cocoa, w/low-fat milk | 1 |
| Milk, evaporated, skim | 1 |
| Yoo-Hoo, chocolate drink | 1 |
| Coffees, flavored, sugar-free | 3 |
| Milk, low-fat,1% | 3 |
| Slim Fast, most flav, 11 fl oz | 3 |
| Coffees, flavored, reg | 4 |
| Milk, chocolate, low-fat, 2% | 5 |
| Milk, low-fat, 2% | 5 |
| Soy milk | 5 |
| Shake, chocolate, thick | 6 |
| Shake, vanilla, thick | 7 |
| Milk, chocolate, regular | 8 |
| Milk, whole | 8 |
| Cocoa, w/whole milk | 9 |
| Eggnog | 19 |
| Milk, evaporated | 19 |

* Counts for non-alcoholic drinks and beer are based on
  8-fluid-ounce servings, for wine on 3 1/2-fluid-ounce
  servings and, for hard liquor, on 1 1/2-fluid-ounce servings.

86

## Bread, Crackers, Flours:
## BAGELS*

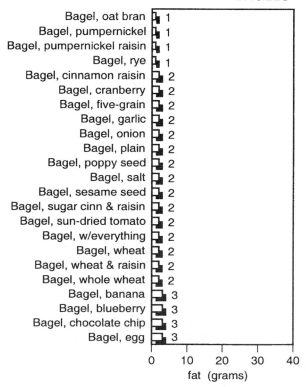

| Bagel, oat bran | 1 |
| Bagel, pumpernickel | 1 |
| Bagel, pumpernickel raisin | 1 |
| Bagel, rye | 1 |
| Bagel, cinnamon raisin | 2 |
| Bagel, cranberry | 2 |
| Bagel, five-grain | 2 |
| Bagel, garlic | 2 |
| Bagel, onion | 2 |
| Bagel, plain | 2 |
| Bagel, poppy seed | 2 |
| Bagel, salt | 2 |
| Bagel, sesame seed | 2 |
| Bagel, sugar cinn & raisin | 2 |
| Bagel, sun-dried tomato | 2 |
| Bagel, w/everything | 2 |
| Bagel, wheat | 2 |
| Bagel, wheat & raisin | 2 |
| Bagel, whole wheat | 2 |
| Bagel, banana | 3 |
| Bagel, blueberry | 3 |
| Bagel, chocolate chip | 3 |
| Bagel, egg | 3 |

fat (grams)

\* Counts are based on one bagel, approximate weight:
3 ounces.

## Bread, Crackers, and Flour:
## BISCUITS, ROLLS & MUFFINS*

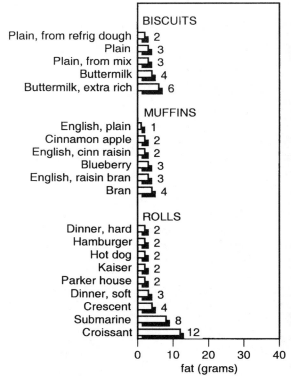

BISCUITS

| | |
|---|---|
| Plain, from refrig dough | 2 |
| Plain | 3 |
| Plain, from mix | 3 |
| Buttermilk | 4 |
| Buttermilk, extra rich | 6 |

MUFFINS

| | |
|---|---|
| English, plain | 1 |
| Cinnamon apple | 2 |
| English, cinn raisin | 2 |
| Blueberry | 3 |
| English, raisin bran | 3 |
| Bran | 4 |

ROLLS

| | |
|---|---|
| Dinner, hard | 2 |
| Hamburger | 2 |
| Hot dog | 2 |
| Kaiser | 2 |
| Parker house | 2 |
| Dinner, soft | 3 |
| Crescent | 4 |
| Submarine | 8 |
| Croissant | 12 |

0    10    20    30    40
fat (grams)

* Counts are based on single, average-size items. Average
sweet muffin is assumed to be 2 3/4 inches by 2 inches.
Average sweet and English muffin weight is 57 grams.

88

## Bread, Crackers, and Flours: BREAD*

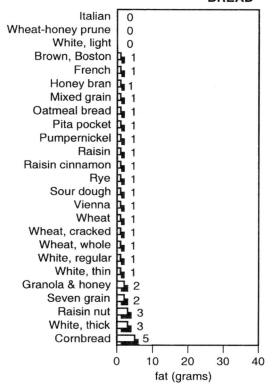

| | fat (grams) |
|---|---|
| Italian | 0 |
| Wheat-honey prune | 0 |
| White, light | 0 |
| Brown, Boston | 1 |
| French | 1 |
| Honey bran | 1 |
| Mixed grain | 1 |
| Oatmeal bread | 1 |
| Pita pocket | 1 |
| Pumpernickel | 1 |
| Raisin | 1 |
| Raisin cinnamon | 1 |
| Rye | 1 |
| Sour dough | 1 |
| Vienna | 1 |
| Wheat | 1 |
| Wheat, cracked | 1 |
| Wheat, whole | 1 |
| White, regular | 1 |
| White, thin | 1 |
| Granola & honey | 2 |
| Seven grain | 2 |
| Raisin nut | 3 |
| White, thick | 3 |
| Cornbread | 5 |

fat (grams)

\* Counts are based on single, average-size slices.

89

Hi-Low Comparison Chart
(for Alphabetical Charts, see pages 1 - 82)

## Bread, Crackers, and Flours: CRACKERS*

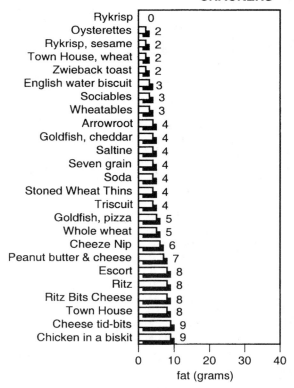

| Cracker | fat (grams) |
|---|---|
| Rykrisp | 0 |
| Oysterettes | 2 |
| Rykrisp, sesame | 2 |
| Town House, wheat | 2 |
| Zwieback toast | 2 |
| English water biscuit | 3 |
| Sociables | 3 |
| Wheatables | 3 |
| Arrowroot | 4 |
| Goldfish, cheddar | 4 |
| Saltine | 4 |
| Seven grain | 4 |
| Soda | 4 |
| Stoned Wheat Thins | 4 |
| Triscuit | 4 |
| Goldfish, pizza | 5 |
| Whole wheat | 5 |
| Cheeze Nip | 6 |
| Peanut butter & cheese | 7 |
| Escort | 8 |
| Ritz | 8 |
| Ritz Bits Cheese | 8 |
| Town House | 8 |
| Cheese tid-bits | 9 |
| Chicken in a biskit | 9 |

\* For ease of comparison, counts are based on one-ounce servings. Adjust counts to reflect quantities consumed.

## Bread, Crackers, and Flours:
## DRY & CRISPY*

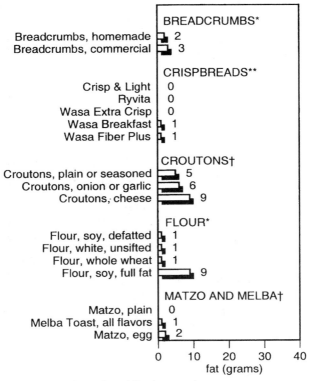

BREADCRUMBS*

Breadcrumbs, homemade 2
Breadcrumbs, commercial 3

CRISPBREADS**

Crisp & Light 0
Ryvita 0
Wasa Extra Crisp 0
Wasa Breakfast 1
Wasa Fiber Plus 1

CROUTONS†

Croutons, plain or seasoned 5
Croutons, onion or garlic 6
Croutons, cheese 9

FLOUR*

Flour, soy, defatted 1
Flour, white, unsifted 1
Flour, whole wheat 1
Flour, soy, full fat 9

MATZO AND MELBA†

Matzo, plain 0
Melba Toast, all flavors 1
Matzo, egg 2

0   10   20   30   40
fat (grams)

\* Counts are based on 1/2- cup servings.

\*\* Counts are based on single item.

† Counts are based on single-ounce servings.

## Bread, Crackers, and Flours:
## PANCAKES, STUFFING & MORE*

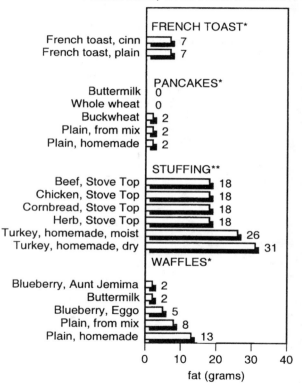

FRENCH TOAST*

French toast, cinn — 7
French toast, plain — 7

PANCAKES*

Buttermilk 0
Whole wheat 0
Buckwheat — 2
Plain, from mix — 2
Plain, homemade — 2

STUFFING**

Beef, Stove Top — 18
Chicken, Stove Top — 18
Cornbread, Stove Top — 18
Herb, Stove Top — 18
Turkey, homemade, moist — 26
Turkey, homemade, dry — 31

WAFFLES*

Blueberry, Aunt Jemima — 2
Buttermilk — 2
Blueberry, Eggo — 5
Plain, from mix — 8
Plain, homemade — 13

0    10    20    30    40
fat (grams)

*   Counts are based on single slice, pancake, or waffle.
**  Counts are based on 1/2-cup servings, prepared.

## CEREALS*, Part 1

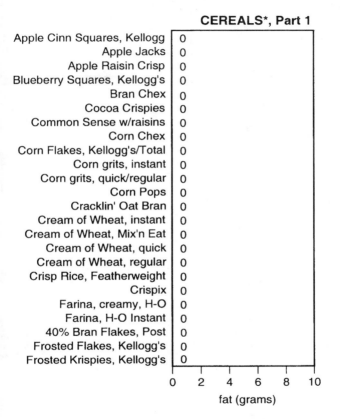

| | fat (grams) |
|---|---|
| Apple Cinn Squares, Kellogg | 0 |
| Apple Jacks | 0 |
| Apple Raisin Crisp | 0 |
| Blueberry Squares, Kellogg's | 0 |
| Bran Chex | 0 |
| Cocoa Crispies | 0 |
| Common Sense w/raisins | 0 |
| Corn Chex | 0 |
| Corn Flakes, Kellogg's/Total | 0 |
| Corn grits, instant | 0 |
| Corn grits, quick/regular | 0 |
| Corn Pops | 0 |
| Cracklin' Oat Bran | 0 |
| Cream of Wheat, instant | 0 |
| Cream of Wheat, Mix'n Eat | 0 |
| Cream of Wheat, quick | 0 |
| Cream of Wheat, regular | 0 |
| Crisp Rice, Featherweight | 0 |
| Crispix | 0 |
| Farina, creamy, H-O | 0 |
| Farina, H-O Instant | 0 |
| 40% Bran Flakes, Post | 0 |
| Frosted Flakes, Kellogg's | 0 |
| Frosted Krispies, Kellogg's | 0 |

0   2   4   6   8   10

fat (grams)

* Counts are based on average-size servings (as indicated
on package) and without added milk.

**CEREALS\*, Part 2**

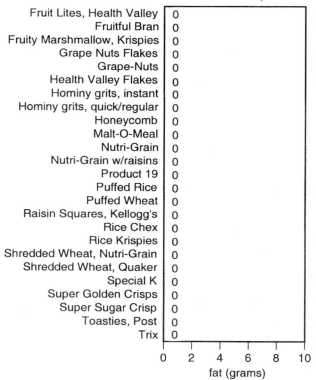

| | fat (grams) |
|---|---|
| Fruit Lites, Health Valley | 0 |
| Fruitful Bran | 0 |
| Fruity Marshmallow, Krispies | 0 |
| Grape Nuts Flakes | 0 |
| Grape-Nuts | 0 |
| Health Valley Flakes | 0 |
| Hominy grits, instant | 0 |
| Hominy grits, quick/regular | 0 |
| Honeycomb | 0 |
| Malt-O-Meal | 0 |
| Nutri-Grain | 0 |
| Nutri-Grain w/raisins | 0 |
| Product 19 | 0 |
| Puffed Rice | 0 |
| Puffed Wheat | 0 |
| Raisin Squares, Kellogg's | 0 |
| Rice Chex | 0 |
| Rice Krispies | 0 |
| Shredded Wheat, Nutri-Grain | 0 |
| Shredded Wheat, Quaker | 0 |
| Special K | 0 |
| Super Golden Crisps | 0 |
| Super Sugar Crisp | 0 |
| Toasties, Post | 0 |
| Trix | 0 |

\* Counts are based on average-size servings (as indicated on package) and without added milk.

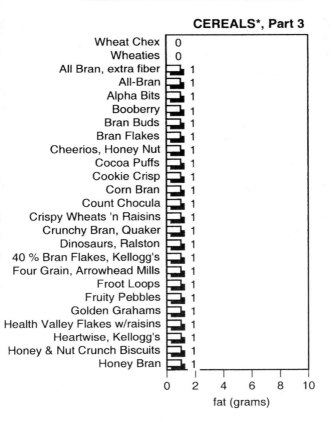

## Hi-Low Comparison Chart
(for Alphabetical Charts, see pages 1 - 82)

### CEREALS*, Part 3

| | fat (grams) |
|---|---|
| Wheat Chex | 0 |
| Wheaties | 0 |
| All Bran, extra fiber | 1 |
| All-Bran | 1 |
| Alpha Bits | 1 |
| Booberry | 1 |
| Bran Buds | 1 |
| Bran Flakes | 1 |
| Cheerios, Honey Nut | 1 |
| Cocoa Puffs | 1 |
| Cookie Crisp | 1 |
| Corn Bran | 1 |
| Count Chocula | 1 |
| Crispy Wheats 'n Raisins | 1 |
| Crunchy Bran, Quaker | 1 |
| Dinosaurs, Ralston | 1 |
| 40 % Bran Flakes, Kellogg's | 1 |
| Four Grain, Arrowhead Mills | 1 |
| Froot Loops | 1 |
| Fruity Pebbles | 1 |
| Golden Grahams | 1 |
| Health Valley Flakes w/raisins | 1 |
| Heartwise, Kellogg's | 1 |
| Honey & Nut Crunch Biscuits | 1 |
| Honey Bran | 1 |

0   2   4   6   8   10
fat (grams)

\* Counts are based on average-size servings (as indicated
on package) and without added milk.

## CEREALS*, Part 4

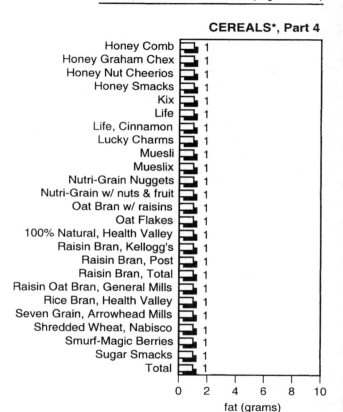

| | fat (grams) |
|---|---|
| Honey Comb | 1 |
| Honey Graham Chex | 1 |
| Honey Nut Cheerios | 1 |
| Honey Smacks | 1 |
| Kix | 1 |
| Life | 1 |
| Life, Cinnamon | 1 |
| Lucky Charms | 1 |
| Muesli | 1 |
| Mueslix | 1 |
| Nutri-Grain Nuggets | 1 |
| Nutri-Grain w/ nuts & fruit | 1 |
| Oat Bran w/ raisins | 1 |
| Oat Flakes | 1 |
| 100% Natural, Health Valley | 1 |
| Raisin Bran, Kellogg's | 1 |
| Raisin Bran, Post | 1 |
| Raisin Bran, Total | 1 |
| Raisin Oat Bran, General Mills | 1 |
| Rice Bran, Health Valley | 1 |
| Seven Grain, Arrowhead Mills | 1 |
| Shredded Wheat, Nabisco | 1 |
| Smurf-Magic Berries | 1 |
| Sugar Smacks | 1 |
| Total | 1 |

\* Counts are based on average-size servings (as indicated
on package) and without added milk.

## CEREALS*, Part 5

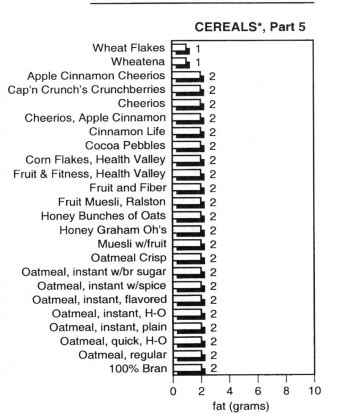

| Cereal | fat (grams) |
|---|---|
| Wheat Flakes | 1 |
| Wheatena | 1 |
| Apple Cinnamon Cheerios | 2 |
| Cap'n Crunch's Crunchberries | 2 |
| Cheerios | 2 |
| Cheerios, Apple Cinnamon | 2 |
| Cinnamon Life | 2 |
| Cocoa Pebbles | 2 |
| Corn Flakes, Health Valley | 2 |
| Fruit & Fitness, Health Valley | 2 |
| Fruit and Fiber | 2 |
| Fruit Muesli, Ralston | 2 |
| Honey Bunches of Oats | 2 |
| Honey Graham Oh's | 2 |
| Muesli w/fruit | 2 |
| Oatmeal Crisp | 2 |
| Oatmeal, instant w/br sugar | 2 |
| Oatmeal, instant w/spice | 2 |
| Oatmeal, instant, flavored | 2 |
| Oatmeal, instant, H-O | 2 |
| Oatmeal, instant, plain | 2 |
| Oatmeal, quick, H-O | 2 |
| Oatmeal, regular | 2 |
| 100% Bran | 2 |

* Counts are based on average-size servings (as indicated
on package) and without added milk.

97

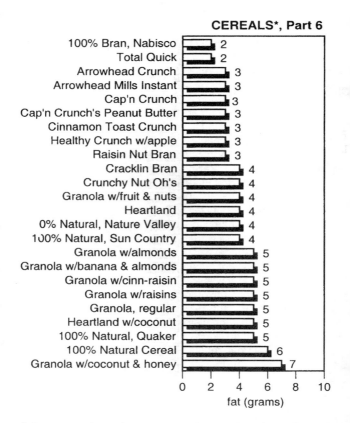

**CEREALS\*, Part 6**

| Cereal | fat (grams) |
|---|---|
| 100% Bran, Nabisco | 2 |
| Total Quick | 2 |
| Arrowhead Crunch | 3 |
| Arrowhead Mills Instant | 3 |
| Cap'n Crunch | 3 |
| Cap'n Crunch's Peanut Butter | 3 |
| Cinnamon Toast Crunch | 3 |
| Healthy Crunch w/apple | 3 |
| Raisin Nut Bran | 3 |
| Cracklin Bran | 4 |
| Crunchy Nut Oh's | 4 |
| Granola w/fruit & nuts | 4 |
| Heartland | 4 |
| 0% Natural, Nature Valley | 4 |
| 100% Natural, Sun Country | 4 |
| Granola w/almonds | 5 |
| Granola w/banana & almonds | 5 |
| Granola w/cinn-raisin | 5 |
| Granola w/raisins | 5 |
| Granola, regular | 5 |
| Heartland w/coconut | 5 |
| 100% Natural, Quaker | 5 |
| 100% Natural Cereal | 6 |
| Granola w/coconut & honey | 7 |

\* Counts are based on average-size servings (as indicated
on package) and without added milk.

## COMBINED AND FROZEN FOODS*,
Part 1

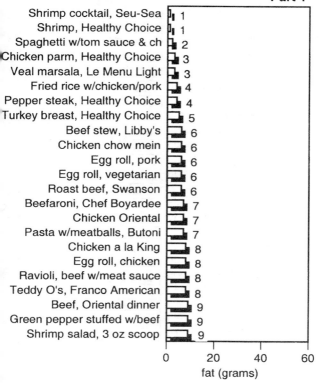

| | fat (grams) |
|---|---|
| Shrimp cocktail, Seu-Sea | 1 |
| Shrimp, Healthy Choice | 1 |
| Spaghetti w/tom sauce & ch | 2 |
| Chicken parm, Healthy Choice | 3 |
| Veal marsala, Le Menu Light | 3 |
| Fried rice w/chicken/pork | 4 |
| Pepper steak, Healthy Choice | 4 |
| Turkey breast, Healthy Choice | 5 |
| Beef stew, Libby's | 6 |
| Chicken chow mein | 6 |
| Egg roll, pork | 6 |
| Egg roll, vegetarian | 6 |
| Roast beef, Swanson | 6 |
| Beefaroni, Chef Boyardee | 7 |
| Chicken Oriental | 7 |
| Pasta w/meatballs, Butoni | 7 |
| Chicken a la King | 8 |
| Egg roll, chicken | 8 |
| Ravioli, beef w/meat sauce | 8 |
| Teddy O's, Franco American | 8 |
| Beef, Oriental dinner | 9 |
| Green pepper stuffed w/beef | 9 |
| Shrimp salad, 3 oz scoop | 9 |

0   20   40   60
fat (grams)

\* Counts are based on average-size servings as indicated
on package. Adjust count to reflect amount consumed.

## COMBINED AND FROZEN FOODS*,
### Part 2

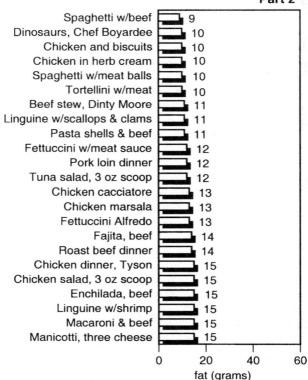

| Food | fat (grams) |
|------|-------------|
| Spaghetti w/beef | 9 |
| Dinosaurs, Chef Boyardee | 10 |
| Chicken and biscuits | 10 |
| Chicken in herb cream | 10 |
| Spaghetti w/meat balls | 10 |
| Tortellini w/meat | 10 |
| Beef stew, Dinty Moore | 11 |
| Linguine w/scallops & clams | 11 |
| Pasta shells & beef | 11 |
| Fettuccini w/meat sauce | 12 |
| Pork loin dinner | 12 |
| Tuna salad, 3 oz scoop | 12 |
| Chicken cacciatore | 13 |
| Chicken marsala | 13 |
| Fettuccini Alfredo | 13 |
| Fajita, beef | 14 |
| Roast beef dinner | 14 |
| Chicken dinner, Tyson | 15 |
| Chicken salad, 3 oz scoop | 15 |
| Enchilada, beef | 15 |
| Linguine w/shrimp | 15 |
| Macaroni & beef | 15 |
| Manicotti, three cheese | 15 |

0    20    40    60
fat (grams)

\* Counts are based on average-size servings as indicated
on package. Adjust count to reflect amount consumed.

Hi-Low Comparison Chart
(for Alphabetical Charts, see pages 1 - 82)

## COMBINED AND FROZEN FOODS*,
### Part 3

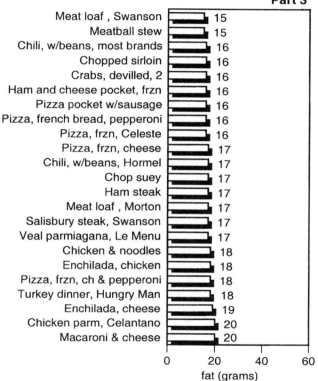

| Food | fat (grams) |
|------|-------------|
| Meat loaf , Swanson | 15 |
| Meatball stew | 15 |
| Chili, w/beans, most brands | 16 |
| Chopped sirloin | 16 |
| Crabs, devilled, 2 | 16 |
| Ham and cheese pocket, frzn | 16 |
| Pizza pocket w/sausage | 16 |
| Pizza, french bread, pepperoni | 16 |
| Pizza, frzn, Celeste | 16 |
| Pizza, frzn, cheese | 17 |
| Chili, w/beans, Hormel | 17 |
| Chop suey | 17 |
| Ham steak | 17 |
| Meat loaf , Morton | 17 |
| Salisbury steak, Swanson | 17 |
| Veal parmiagana, Le Menu | 17 |
| Chicken & noodles | 18 |
| Enchilada, chicken | 18 |
| Pizza, frzn, ch & pepperoni | 18 |
| Turkey dinner, Hungry Man | 18 |
| Enchilada, cheese | 19 |
| Chicken parm, Celentano | 20 |
| Macaroni & cheese | 20 |

* Counts are based on average-size servings as indicated
on package. Adjust count to reflect amount consumed.

101

## COMBINED AND FROZEN FOODS*,
## Part 4

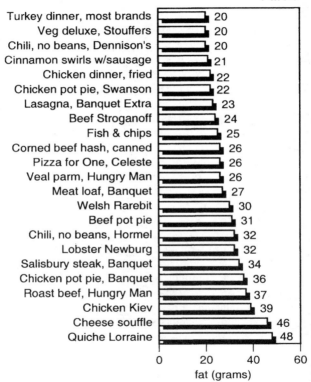

| Food | fat (grams) |
|------|-------------|
| Turkey dinner, most brands | 20 |
| Veg deluxe, Stouffers | 20 |
| Chili, no beans, Dennison's | 20 |
| Cinnamon swirls w/sausage | 21 |
| Chicken dinner, fried | 22 |
| Chicken pot pie, Swanson | 22 |
| Lasagna, Banquet Extra | 23 |
| Beef Stroganoff | 24 |
| Fish & chips | 25 |
| Corned beef hash, canned | 26 |
| Pizza for One, Celeste | 26 |
| Veal parm, Hungry Man | 26 |
| Meat loaf, Banquet | 27 |
| Welsh Rarebit | 30 |
| Beef pot pie | 31 |
| Chili, no beans, Hormel | 32 |
| Lobster Newburg | 32 |
| Salisbury steak, Banquet | 34 |
| Chicken pot pie, Banquet | 36 |
| Roast beef, Hungry Man | 37 |
| Chicken Kiev | 39 |
| Cheese souffle | 46 |
| Quiche Lorraine | 48 |

* Counts are based on average-size servings as indicated
on package. Adjust count to reflect amount consumed.

102

## Dairy: CHEESE (HARD & SEMI-SOFT)*

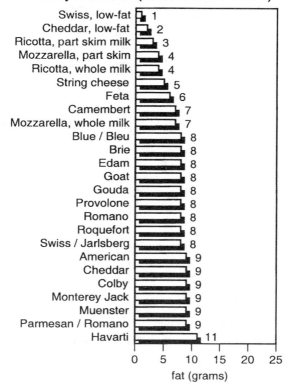

| Cheese | fat (grams) |
|---|---|
| Swiss, low-fat | 1 |
| Cheddar, low-fat | 2 |
| Ricotta, part skim milk | 3 |
| Mozzarella, part skim | 4 |
| Ricotta, whole milk | 4 |
| String cheese | 5 |
| Feta | 6 |
| Camembert | 7 |
| Mozzarella, whole milk | 7 |
| Blue / Bleu | 8 |
| Brie | 8 |
| Edam | 8 |
| Goat | 8 |
| Gouda | 8 |
| Provolone | 8 |
| Romano | 8 |
| Roquefort | 8 |
| Swiss / Jarlsberg | 8 |
| American | 9 |
| Cheddar | 9 |
| Colby | 9 |
| Monterey Jack | 9 |
| Muenster | 9 |
| Parmesan / Romano | 9 |
| Havarti | 11 |

* Counts are based on one-ounce servings. Adjust count
to reflect amount consumed.

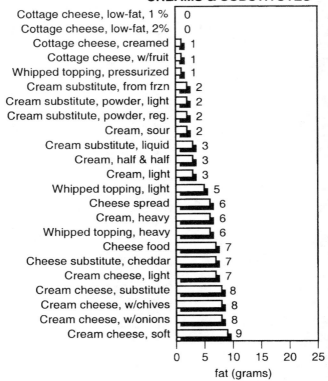

## Dairy: CHEESES (SOFT), CREAMS & SUBSTITUTES*

| Food | fat (grams) |
|------|-------------|
| Cottage cheese, low-fat, 1 % | 0 |
| Cottage cheese, low-fat, 2% | 0 |
| Cottage cheese, creamed | 1 |
| Cottage cheese, w/fruit | 1 |
| Whipped topping, pressurized | 1 |
| Cream substitute, from frzn | 2 |
| Cream substitute, powder, light | 2 |
| Cream substitute, powder, reg. | 2 |
| Cream, sour | 2 |
| Cream substitute, liquid | 3 |
| Cream, half & half | 3 |
| Cream, light | 3 |
| Whipped topping, light | 5 |
| Cheese spread | 6 |
| Cream, heavy | 6 |
| Whipped topping, heavy | 6 |
| Cheese food | 7 |
| Cheese substitute, cheddar | 7 |
| Cream cheese, light | 7 |
| Cream cheese, substitute | 8 |
| Cream cheese, w/chives | 8 |
| Cream cheese, w/onions | 8 |
| Cream cheese, soft | 9 |

* Counts are based on one-ounce servings of soft cheese
or one tablespoon of cream or whipped topping.

104

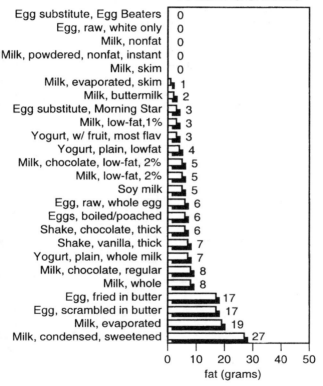

Hi-Low Comparison Chart
(for Alphabetical Charts, see pages 1 - 82)

**Dairy: EGGS, MILK,
YOGURT & SHAKES***

| | fat (grams) |
|---|---|
| Egg substitute, Egg Beaters | 0 |
| Egg, raw, white only | 0 |
| Milk, nonfat | 0 |
| Milk, powdered, nonfat, instant | 0 |
| Milk, skim | 0 |
| Milk, evaporated, skim | 1 |
| Milk, buttermilk | 2 |
| Egg substitute, Morning Star | 3 |
| Milk, low-fat,1% | 3 |
| Yogurt, w/ fruit, most flav | 3 |
| Yogurt, plain, lowfat | 4 |
| Milk, chocolate, low-fat, 2% | 5 |
| Milk, low-fat, 2% | 5 |
| Soy milk | 5 |
| Egg, raw, whole egg | 6 |
| Eggs, boiled/poached | 6 |
| Shake, chocolate, thick | 6 |
| Shake, vanilla, thick | 7 |
| Yogurt, plain, whole milk | 7 |
| Milk, chocolate, regular | 8 |
| Milk, whole | 8 |
| Egg, fried in butter | 17 |
| Egg, scrambled in butter | 17 |
| Milk, evaporated | 19 |
| Milk, condensed, sweetened | 27 |

0    10    20    30    40    50
fat (grams)

* Counts based on one egg or equivalent egg substitute or 8 fluid ounces of milk, yogurt, or shake.

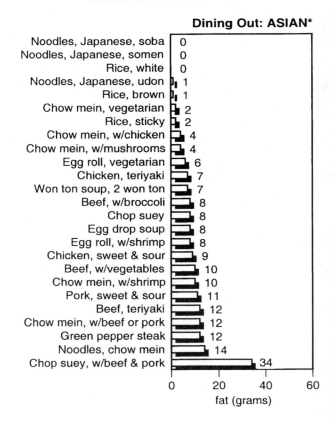

**Dining Out: ASIAN***

| | fat (grams) |
|---|---|
| Noodles, Japanese, soba | 0 |
| Noodles, Japanese, somen | 0 |
| Rice, white | 0 |
| Noodles, Japanese, udon | 1 |
| Rice, brown | 1 |
| Chow mein, vegetarian | 2 |
| Rice, sticky | 2 |
| Chow mein, w/chicken | 4 |
| Chow mein, w/mushrooms | 4 |
| Egg roll, vegetarian | 6 |
| Chicken, teriyaki | 7 |
| Won ton soup, 2 won ton | 7 |
| Beef, w/broccoli | 8 |
| Chop suey | 8 |
| Egg drop soup | 8 |
| Egg roll, w/shrimp | 8 |
| Chicken, sweet & sour | 9 |
| Beef, w/vegetables | 10 |
| Chow mein, w/shrimp | 10 |
| Pork, sweet & sour | 11 |
| Beef, teriyaki | 12 |
| Chow mein, w/beef or pork | 12 |
| Green pepper steak | 12 |
| Noodles, chow mein | 14 |
| Chop suey, w/beef & pork | 34 |

* Counts based on average-sized servings (for main dishes,
1 1/2 - 2 cups). Counts for main dishes include rice.

**Dining Out: DELICATESSEN***

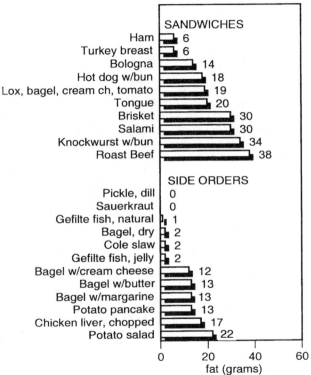

SANDWICHES

| | |
|---|---|
| Ham | 6 |
| Turkey breast | 6 |
| Bologna | 14 |
| Hot dog w/bun | 18 |
| Lox, bagel, cream ch, tomato | 19 |
| Tongue | 20 |
| Brisket | 30 |
| Salami | 30 |
| Knockwurst w/bun | 34 |
| Roast Beef | 38 |

SIDE ORDERS

| | |
|---|---|
| Pickle, dill | 0 |
| Sauerkraut | 0 |
| Gefilte fish, natural | 1 |
| Bagel, dry | 2 |
| Cole slaw | 2 |
| Gefilte fish, jelly | 2 |
| Bagel w/cream cheese | 12 |
| Bagel w/butter | 13 |
| Bagel w/margarine | 13 |
| Potato pancake | 13 |
| Chicken liver, chopped | 17 |
| Potato salad | 22 |

0    20    40    60
fat (grams)

\* Unless otherwise indicated, counts based on average-
size servings or sandwiches. Sandwich counts assume
white or rye bread.

## Dining Out: FRENCH AND OTHER INTERNATIONAL DISHES*

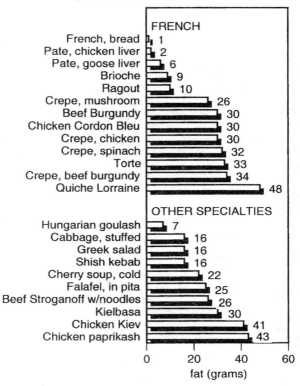

FRENCH

| Dish | fat (grams) |
|------|-------------|
| French, bread | 1 |
| Pate, chicken liver | 2 |
| Pate, goose liver | 6 |
| Brioche | 9 |
| Ragout | 10 |
| Crepe, mushroom | 26 |
| Beef Burgundy | 30 |
| Chicken Cordon Bleu | 30 |
| Crepe, chicken | 30 |
| Crepe, spinach | 32 |
| Torte | 33 |
| Crepe, beef burgundy | 34 |
| Quiche Lorraine | 48 |

OTHER SPECIALTIES

| Dish | fat (grams) |
|------|-------------|
| Hungarian goulash | 7 |
| Cabbage, stuffed | 16 |
| Greek salad | 16 |
| Shish kebab | 16 |
| Cherry soup, cold | 22 |
| Falafel, in pita | 25 |
| Beef Stroganoff w/noodles | 26 |
| Kielbasa | 30 |
| Chicken Kiev | 41 |
| Chicken paprikash | 43 |

fat (grams)

\* Counts based on average-sized servings (for main dishes,
1 1/2 - 2 cups).

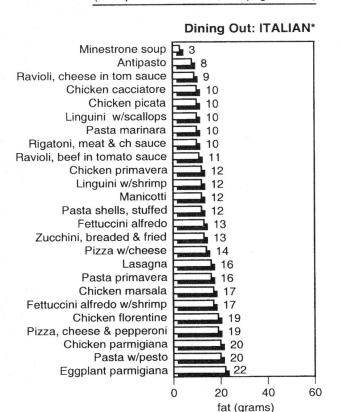

## Hi-Low Comparison Chart
(for Alphabetical Charts, see pages 1 - 82)

**Dining Out: ITALIAN\***

| Item | fat (grams) |
|---|---|
| Minestrone soup | 3 |
| Antipasto | 8 |
| Ravioli, cheese in tom sauce | 9 |
| Chicken cacciatore | 10 |
| Chicken picata | 10 |
| Linguini w/scallops | 10 |
| Pasta marinara | 10 |
| Rigatoni, meat & ch sauce | 10 |
| Ravioli, beef in tomato sauce | 11 |
| Chicken primavera | 12 |
| Linguini w/shrimp | 12 |
| Manicotti | 12 |
| Pasta shells, stuffed | 12 |
| Fettuccini alfredo | 13 |
| Zucchini, breaded & fried | 13 |
| Pizza w/cheese | 14 |
| Lasagna | 16 |
| Pasta primavera | 16 |
| Chicken marsala | 17 |
| Fettuccini alfredo w/shrimp | 17 |
| Chicken florentine | 19 |
| Pizza, cheese & pepperoni | 19 |
| Chicken parmigiana | 20 |
| Pasta w/pesto | 20 |
| Eggplant parmigiana | 22 |

\* Counts are based on average-sized servings (1 1/2 - 2 cups); for pizza, on 1/6 medium or 1/8 large pizza).

**Dining Out: MEXICAN\***

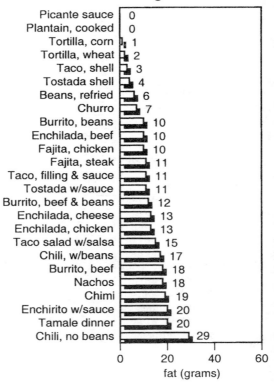

| Food | fat (grams) |
|---|---|
| Picante sauce | 0 |
| Plantain, cooked | 0 |
| Tortilla, corn | 1 |
| Tortilla, wheat | 2 |
| Taco, shell | 3 |
| Tostada shell | 4 |
| Beans, refried | 6 |
| Churro | 7 |
| Burrito, beans | 10 |
| Enchilada, beef | 10 |
| Fajita, chicken | 10 |
| Fajita, steak | 11 |
| Taco, filling & sauce | 11 |
| Tostada w/sauce | 11 |
| Burrito, beef & beans | 12 |
| Enchilada, cheese | 13 |
| Enchilada, chicken | 13 |
| Taco salad w/salsa | 15 |
| Chili, w/beans | 17 |
| Burrito, beef | 18 |
| Nachos | 18 |
| Chimi | 19 |
| Enchirito w/sauce | 20 |
| Tamale dinner | 20 |
| Chili, no beans | 29 |

\* Counts based on average-sized servings (for main dishes,
1 1/2 - 2 cups).

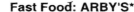

## Hi-Low Comparison Chart
(for Alphabetical Charts, see pages 1 - 82)

**Fast Food: ARBY'S\***

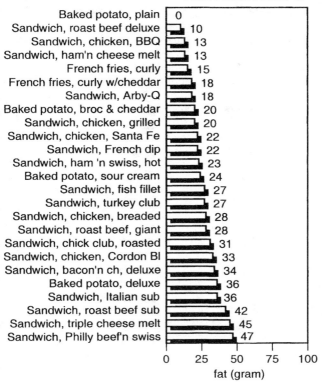

| Item | fat (gram) |
|------|-----------|
| Baked potato, plain | 0 |
| Sandwich, roast beef deluxe | 10 |
| Sandwich, chicken, BBQ | 13 |
| Sandwich, ham'n cheese melt | 13 |
| French fries, curly | 15 |
| French fries, curly w/cheddar | 18 |
| Sandwich, Arby-Q | 18 |
| Baked potato, broc & cheddar | 20 |
| Sandwich, chicken, grilled | 20 |
| Sandwich, chicken, Santa Fe | 22 |
| Sandwich, French dip | 22 |
| Sandwich, ham 'n swiss, hot | 23 |
| Baked potato, sour cream | 24 |
| Sandwich, fish fillet | 27 |
| Sandwich, turkey club | 27 |
| Sandwich, chicken, breaded | 28 |
| Sandwich, roast beef, giant | 28 |
| Sandwich, chick club, roasted | 31 |
| Sandwich, chicken, Cordon Bl | 33 |
| Sandwich, bacon'n ch, deluxe | 34 |
| Baked potato, deluxe | 36 |
| Sandwich, Italian sub | 36 |
| Sandwich, roast beef sub | 42 |
| Sandwich, triple cheese melt | 45 |
| Sandwich, Philly beef'n swiss | 47 |

fat (gram)

\* Unless otherwise indicated, counts are based on average-size servings.

111

## Fast Food: BOSTON MARKET*

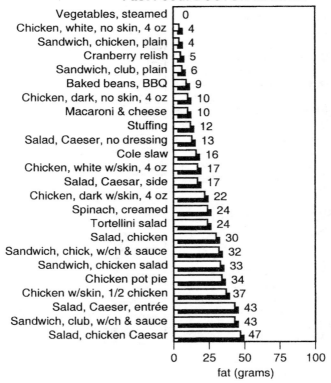

| Food | fat (grams) |
|---|---|
| Vegetables, steamed | 0 |
| Chicken, white, no skin, 4 oz | 4 |
| Sandwich, chicken, plain | 4 |
| Cranberry relish | 5 |
| Sandwich, club, plain | 6 |
| Baked beans, BBQ | 9 |
| Chicken, dark, no skin, 4 oz | 10 |
| Macaroni & cheese | 10 |
| Stuffing | 12 |
| Salad, Caeser, no dressing | 13 |
| Cole slaw | 16 |
| Chicken, white w/skin, 4 oz | 17 |
| Salad, Caesar, side | 17 |
| Chicken, dark w/skin, 4 oz | 22 |
| Spinach, creamed | 24 |
| Tortellini salad | 24 |
| Salad, chicken | 30 |
| Sandwich, chick, w/ch & sauce | 32 |
| Sandwich, chicken salad | 33 |
| Chicken pot pie | 34 |
| Chicken w/skin, 1/2 chicken | 37 |
| Salad, Caeser, entrée | 43 |
| Sandwich, club, w/ch & sauce | 43 |
| Salad, chicken Caesar | 47 |

* Unless otherwise indicated, counts are based on average-size servings.

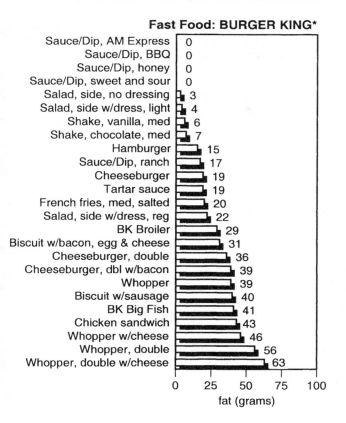

Hi-Low Comparison Chart
(for Alphabetical Charts, see pages 1 - 82)

## Fast Food: BURGER KING*

| Item | fat (grams) |
|------|-------------|
| Sauce/Dip, AM Express | 0 |
| Sauce/Dip, BBQ | 0 |
| Sauce/Dip, honey | 0 |
| Sauce/Dip, sweet and sour | 0 |
| Salad, side, no dressing | 3 |
| Salad, side w/dress, light | 4 |
| Shake, vanilla, med | 6 |
| Shake, chocolate, med | 7 |
| Hamburger | 15 |
| Sauce/Dip, ranch | 17 |
| Cheeseburger | 19 |
| Tartar sauce | 19 |
| French fries, med, salted | 20 |
| Salad, side w/dress, reg | 22 |
| BK Broiler | 29 |
| Biscuit w/bacon, egg & cheese | 31 |
| Cheeseburger, double | 36 |
| Cheeseburger, dbl w/bacon | 39 |
| Whopper | 39 |
| Biscuit w/sausage | 40 |
| BK Big Fish | 41 |
| Chicken sandwich | 43 |
| Whopper w/cheese | 46 |
| Whopper, double | 56 |
| Whopper, double w/cheese | 63 |

fat (grams): 0   25   50   75   100

* Unless otherwise indicated, counts are based on average-size servings.

**Fast Food: HARDEE'S***

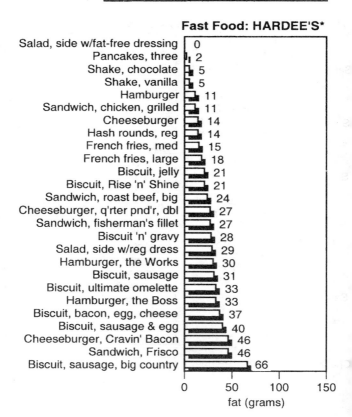

| | fat (grams) |
|---|---|
| Salad, side w/fat-free dressing | 0 |
| Pancakes, three | 2 |
| Shake, chocolate | 5 |
| Shake, vanilla | 5 |
| Hamburger | 11 |
| Sandwich, chicken, grilled | 11 |
| Cheeseburger | 14 |
| Hash rounds, reg | 14 |
| French fries, med | 15 |
| French fries, large | 18 |
| Biscuit, jelly | 21 |
| Biscuit, Rise 'n' Shine | 21 |
| Sandwich, roast beef, big | 24 |
| Cheeseburger, q'rter pnd'r, dbl | 27 |
| Sandwich, fisherman's fillet | 27 |
| Biscuit 'n' gravy | 28 |
| Salad, side w/reg dress | 29 |
| Hamburger, the Works | 30 |
| Biscuit, sausage | 31 |
| Biscuit, ultimate omelette | 33 |
| Hamburger, the Boss | 33 |
| Biscuit, bacon, egg, cheese | 37 |
| Biscuit, sausage & egg | 40 |
| Cheeseburger, Cravin' Bacon | 46 |
| Sandwich, Frisco | 46 |
| Biscuit, sausage, big country | 66 |

* Unless otherwise indicated, counts are based on average-size servings.

114

## Fast Food: JACK IN THE BOX*

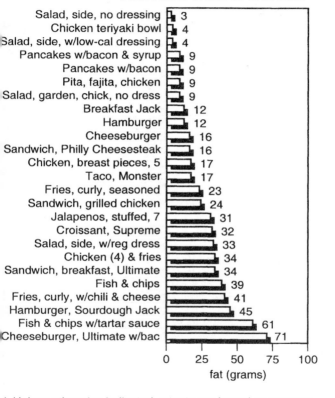

| Item | fat (grams) |
|------|-------------|
| Salad, side, no dressing | 3 |
| Chicken teriyaki bowl | 4 |
| Salad, side, w/low-cal dressing | 4 |
| Pancakes w/bacon & syrup | 9 |
| Pancakes w/bacon | 9 |
| Pita, fajita, chicken | 9 |
| Salad, garden, chick, no dress | 9 |
| Breakfast Jack | 12 |
| Hamburger | 12 |
| Cheeseburger | 16 |
| Sandwich, Philly Cheesesteak | 16 |
| Chicken, breast pieces, 5 | 17 |
| Taco, Monster | 17 |
| Fries, curly, seasoned | 23 |
| Sandwich, grilled chicken | 24 |
| Jalapenos, stuffed, 7 | 31 |
| Croissant, Supreme | 32 |
| Salad, side, w/reg dress | 33 |
| Chicken (4) & fries | 34 |
| Sandwich, breakfast, Ultimate | 34 |
| Fish & chips | 39 |
| Fries, curly, w/chili & cheese | 41 |
| Hamburger, Sourdough Jack | 45 |
| Fish & chips w/tartar sauce | 61 |
| Cheeseburger, Ultimate w/bac | 71 |

* Unless otherwise indicated, counts are based on average-size servings.

**Fast Food: KFC\***

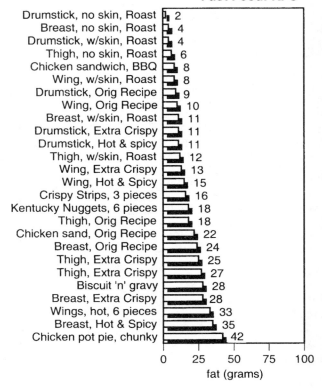

| | fat (grams) |
|---|---|
| Drumstick, no skin, Roast | 2 |
| Breast, no skin, Roast | 4 |
| Drumstick, w/skin, Roast | 4 |
| Thigh, no skin, Roast | 6 |
| Chicken sandwich, BBQ | 8 |
| Wing, w/skin, Roast | 8 |
| Drumstick, Orig Recipe | 9 |
| Wing, Orig Recipe | 10 |
| Breast, w/skin, Roast | 11 |
| Drumstick, Extra Crispy | 11 |
| Drumstick, Hot & spicy | 11 |
| Thigh, w/skin, Roast | 12 |
| Wing, Extra Crispy | 13 |
| Wing, Hot & Spicy | 15 |
| Crispy Strips, 3 pieces | 16 |
| Kentucky Nuggets, 6 pieces | 18 |
| Thigh, Orig Recipe | 18 |
| Chicken sand, Orig Recipe | 22 |
| Breast, Orig Recipe | 24 |
| Thigh, Extra Crispy | 25 |
| Thigh, Extra Crispy | 27 |
| Biscuit 'n' gravy | 28 |
| Breast, Extra Crispy | 28 |
| Wings, hot, 6 pieces | 33 |
| Breast, Hot & Spicy | 35 |
| Chicken pot pie, chunky | 42 |

\* Unless otherwise indicated, counts are based on average-
size servings.

## Fast Food: MC DONALD'S*

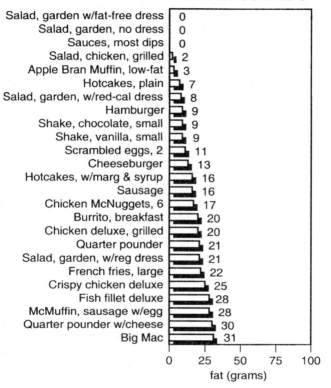

| Item | fat (grams) |
|------|-------------|
| Salad, garden w/fat-free dress | 0 |
| Salad, garden, no dress | 0 |
| Sauces, most dips | 0 |
| Salad, chicken, grilled | 2 |
| Apple Bran Muffin, low-fat | 3 |
| Hotcakes, plain | 7 |
| Salad, garden, w/red-cal dress | 8 |
| Hamburger | 9 |
| Shake, chocolate, small | 9 |
| Shake, vanilla, small | 9 |
| Scrambled eggs, 2 | 11 |
| Cheeseburger | 13 |
| Hotcakes, w/marg & syrup | 16 |
| Sausage | 16 |
| Chicken McNuggets, 6 | 17 |
| Burrito, breakfast | 20 |
| Chicken deluxe, grilled | 20 |
| Quarter pounder | 21 |
| Salad, garden, w/reg dress | 21 |
| French fries, large | 22 |
| Crispy chicken deluxe | 25 |
| Fish fillet deluxe | 28 |
| McMuffin, sausage w/egg | 28 |
| Quarter pounder w/cheese | 30 |
| Big Mac | 31 |

fat (grams)

\* Unless otherwise indicated, counts are based on average-size servings.

**Fast Food: PIZZA HUT\***

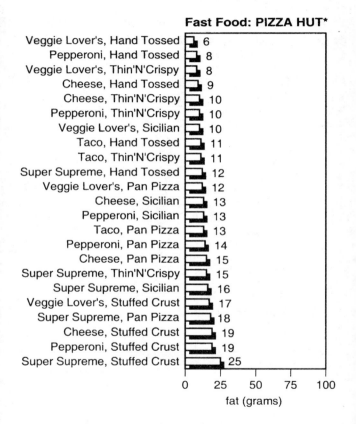

| | fat (grams) |
|---|---|
| Veggie Lover's, Hand Tossed | 6 |
| Pepperoni, Hand Tossed | 8 |
| Veggie Lover's, Thin'N'Crispy | 8 |
| Cheese, Hand Tossed | 9 |
| Cheese, Thin'N'Crispy | 10 |
| Pepperoni, Thin'N'Crispy | 10 |
| Veggie Lover's, Sicilian | 10 |
| Taco, Hand Tossed | 11 |
| Taco, Thin'N'Crispy | 11 |
| Super Supreme, Hand Tossed | 12 |
| Veggie Lover's, Pan Pizza | 12 |
| Cheese, Sicilian | 13 |
| Pepperoni, Sicilian | 13 |
| Taco, Pan Pizza | 13 |
| Pepperoni, Pan Pizza | 14 |
| Cheese, Pan Pizza | 15 |
| Super Supreme, Thin'N'Crispy | 15 |
| Super Supreme, Sicilian | 16 |
| Veggie Lover's, Stuffed Crust | 17 |
| Super Supreme, Pan Pizza | 18 |
| Cheese, Stuffed Crust | 19 |
| Pepperoni, Stuffed Crust | 19 |
| Super Supreme, Stuffed Crust | 25 |

\* Unless otherwise indicated, counts are based on average-
  size servings.

118

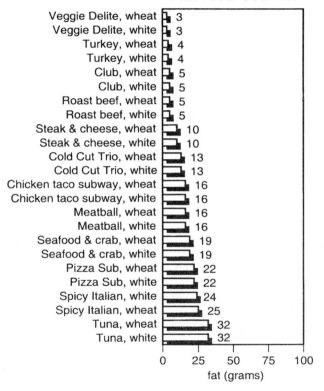

# Hi-Low Comparison Chart
(for Alphabetical Charts, see pages 1 - 82)

## Fast Food: SUBWAY*

| Item | fat (grams) |
|------|-------------|
| Veggie Delite, wheat | 3 |
| Veggie Delite, white | 3 |
| Turkey, wheat | 4 |
| Turkey, white | 4 |
| Club, wheat | 5 |
| Club, white | 5 |
| Roast beef, wheat | 5 |
| Roast beef, white | 5 |
| Steak & cheese, wheat | 10 |
| Steak & cheese, white | 10 |
| Cold Cut Trio, wheat | 13 |
| Cold Cut Trio, white | 13 |
| Chicken taco subway, wheat | 16 |
| Chicken taco subway, white | 16 |
| Meatball, wheat | 16 |
| Meatball, white | 16 |
| Seafood & crab, wheat | 19 |
| Seafood & crab, white | 19 |
| Pizza Sub, wheat | 22 |
| Pizza Sub, white | 22 |
| Spicy Italian, white | 24 |
| Spicy Italian, wheat | 25 |
| Tuna, wheat | 32 |
| Tuna, white | 32 |

fat (grams)

* Unless otherwise indicated, counts are based on average-size servings.

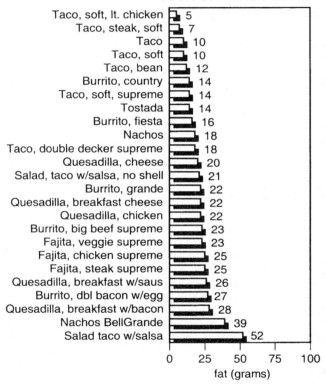

Hi-Low Comparison Chart
(for Alphabetical Charts, see pages 1 - 82)

**Fast Food: TACO BELL\***

| Item | fat (grams) |
|---|---|
| Taco, soft, lt. chicken | 5 |
| Taco, steak, soft | 7 |
| Taco | 10 |
| Taco, soft | 10 |
| Taco, bean | 12 |
| Burrito, country | 14 |
| Taco, soft, supreme | 14 |
| Tostada | 14 |
| Burrito, fiesta | 16 |
| Nachos | 18 |
| Taco, double decker supreme | 18 |
| Quesadilla, cheese | 20 |
| Salad, taco w/salsa, no shell | 21 |
| Burrito, grande | 22 |
| Quesadilla, breakfast cheese | 22 |
| Quesadilla, chicken | 22 |
| Burrito, big beef supreme | 23 |
| Fajita, veggie supreme | 23 |
| Fajita, chicken supreme | 25 |
| Fajita, steak supreme | 25 |
| Quesadilla, breakfast w/saus | 26 |
| Burrito, dbl bacon w/egg | 27 |
| Quesadilla, breakfast w/bacon | 28 |
| Nachos BellGrande | 39 |
| Salad taco w/salsa | 52 |

fat (grams)

\* Unless otherwise indicated, counts are based on average-size servings.

120

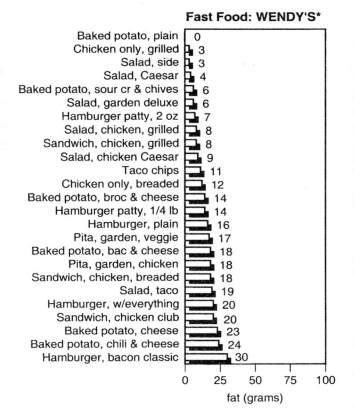

## Hi-Low Comparison Chart
### (for Alphabetical Charts, see pages 1 - 82)

**Fast Food: WENDY'S***

| Item | fat (grams) |
|------|-------------|
| Baked potato, plain | 0 |
| Chicken only, grilled | 3 |
| Salad, side | 3 |
| Salad, Caesar | 4 |
| Baked potato, sour cr & chives | 6 |
| Salad, garden deluxe | 6 |
| Hamburger patty, 2 oz | 7 |
| Salad, chicken, grilled | 8 |
| Sandwich, chicken, grilled | 8 |
| Salad, chicken Caesar | 9 |
| Taco chips | 11 |
| Chicken only, breaded | 12 |
| Baked potato, broc & cheese | 14 |
| Hamburger patty, 1/4 lb | 14 |
| Hamburger, plain | 16 |
| Pita, garden, veggie | 17 |
| Baked potato, bac & cheese | 18 |
| Pita, garden, chicken | 18 |
| Sandwich, chicken, breaded | 18 |
| Salad, taco | 19 |
| Hamburger, w/everything | 20 |
| Sandwich, chicken club | 20 |
| Baked potato, cheese | 23 |
| Baked potato, chili & cheese | 24 |
| Hamburger, bacon classic | 30 |

fat (grams) — scale: 0, 25, 50, 75, 100

* Unless otherwise indicated, counts are based on average-size servings.

121

## Fruits: FRESH & DRIED FRUITS AND JUICES *, Part 1

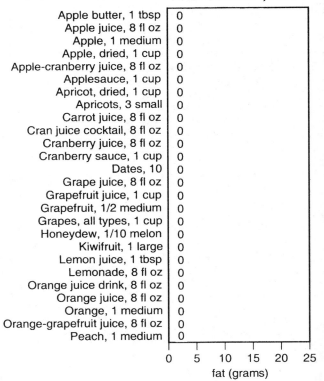

| | fat (grams) |
|---|---|
| Apple butter, 1 tbsp | 0 |
| Apple juice, 8 fl oz | 0 |
| Apple, 1 medium | 0 |
| Apple, dried, 1 cup | 0 |
| Apple-cranberry juice, 8 fl oz | 0 |
| Applesauce, 1 cup | 0 |
| Apricot, dried, 1 cup | 0 |
| Apricots, 3 small | 0 |
| Carrot juice, 8 fl oz | 0 |
| Cran juice cocktail, 8 fl oz | 0 |
| Cranberry juice, 8 fl oz | 0 |
| Cranberry sauce, 1 cup | 0 |
| Dates, 10 | 0 |
| Grape juice, 8 fl oz | 0 |
| Grapefruit juice, 1 cup | 0 |
| Grapefruit, 1/2 medium | 0 |
| Grapes, all types, 1 cup | 0 |
| Honeydew, 1/10 melon | 0 |
| Kiwifruit, 1 large | 0 |
| Lemon juice, 1 tbsp | 0 |
| Lemonade, 8 fl oz | 0 |
| Orange juice drink, 8 fl oz | 0 |
| Orange juice, 8 fl oz | 0 |
| Orange, 1 medium | 0 |
| Orange-grapefruit juice, 8 fl oz | 0 |
| Peach, 1 medium | 0 |

0    5    10    15    20    25
fat (grams)

* Unless otherwise indicated, counts are based on whole, fresh fruits.

122

### Fruits: FRESH & DRIED FRUITS
### AND JUICES *, Part 2

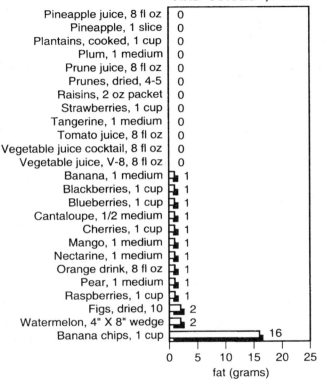

| Food | fat (grams) |
|------|-------------|
| Pineapple juice, 8 fl oz | 0 |
| Pineapple, 1 slice | 0 |
| Plantains, cooked, 1 cup | 0 |
| Plum, 1 medium | 0 |
| Prune juice, 8 fl oz | 0 |
| Prunes, dried, 4-5 | 0 |
| Raisins, 2 oz packet | 0 |
| Strawberries, 1 cup | 0 |
| Tangerine, 1 medium | 0 |
| Tomato juice, 8 fl oz | 0 |
| Vegetable juice cocktail, 8 fl oz | 0 |
| Vegetable juice, V-8, 8 fl oz | 0 |
| Banana, 1 medium | 1 |
| Blackberries, 1 cup | 1 |
| Blueberries, 1 cup | 1 |
| Cantaloupe, 1/2 medium | 1 |
| Cherries, 1 cup | 1 |
| Mango, 1 medium | 1 |
| Nectarine, 1 medium | 1 |
| Orange drink, 8 fl oz | 1 |
| Pear, 1 medium | 1 |
| Raspberries, 1 cup | 1 |
| Figs, dried, 10 | 2 |
| Watermelon, 4" X 8" wedge | 2 |
| Banana chips, 1 cup | 16 |

fat (grams)

* Unless otherwise indicated, counts are based on whole,
fresh fruits.

## GRAVIES, SAUCES & DIPS*

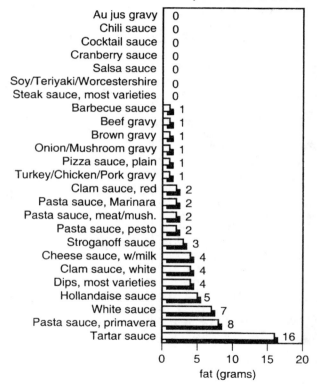

| | fat (grams) |
|---|---|
| Au jus gravy | 0 |
| Chili sauce | 0 |
| Cocktail sauce | 0 |
| Cranberry sauce | 0 |
| Salsa sauce | 0 |
| Soy/Teriyaki/Worcestershire | 0 |
| Steak sauce, most varieties | 0 |
| Barbecue sauce | 1 |
| Beef gravy | 1 |
| Brown gravy | 1 |
| Onion/Mushroom gravy | 1 |
| Pizza sauce, plain | 1 |
| Turkey/Chicken/Pork gravy | 1 |
| Clam sauce, red | 2 |
| Pasta sauce, Marinara | 2 |
| Pasta sauce, meat/mush. | 2 |
| Pasta sauce, pesto | 2 |
| Stroganoff sauce | 3 |
| Cheese sauce, w/milk | 4 |
| Clam sauce, white | 4 |
| Dips, most varieties | 4 |
| Hollandaise sauce | 5 |
| White sauce | 7 |
| Pasta sauce, primavera | 8 |
| Tartar sauce | 16 |

*Counts are based on one-quarter cup servings.

124

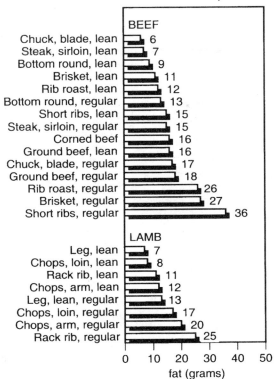

**MEATS\*, Part 1**

BEEF

| | fat (grams) |
|---|---|
| Chuck, blade, lean | 6 |
| Steak, sirloin, lean | 7 |
| Bottom round, lean | 9 |
| Brisket, lean | 11 |
| Rib roast, lean | 12 |
| Bottom round, regular | 13 |
| Short ribs, lean | 15 |
| Steak, sirloin, regular | 15 |
| Corned beef | 16 |
| Ground beef, lean | 16 |
| Chuck, blade, regular | 17 |
| Ground beef, regular | 18 |
| Rib roast, regular | 26 |
| Brisket, regular | 27 |
| Short ribs, regular | 36 |

LAMB

| | fat (grams) |
|---|---|
| Leg, lean | 7 |
| Chops, loin, lean | 8 |
| Rack rib, lean | 11 |
| Chops, arm, lean | 12 |
| Leg, lean, regular | 13 |
| Chops, loin, regular | 17 |
| Chops, arm, regular | 20 |
| Rack rib, regular | 25 |

fat (grams)

\* Counts are based on 3-ounce servings.

## MEATS*, Part 2

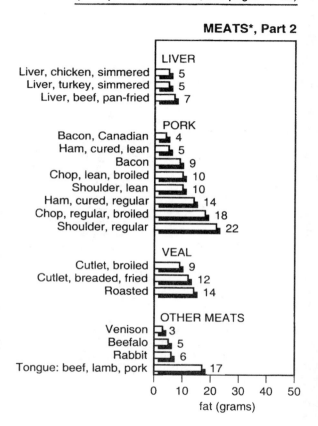

**LIVER**

| | |
|---|---|
| Liver, chicken, simmered | 5 |
| Liver, turkey, simmered | 5 |
| Liver, beef, pan-fried | 7 |

**PORK**

| | |
|---|---|
| Bacon, Canadian | 4 |
| Ham, cured, lean | 5 |
| Bacon | 9 |
| Chop, lean, broiled | 10 |
| Shoulder, lean | 10 |
| Ham, cured, regular | 14 |
| Chop, regular, broiled | 18 |
| Shoulder, regular | 22 |

**VEAL**

| | |
|---|---|
| Cutlet, broiled | 9 |
| Cutlet, breaded, fried | 12 |
| Roasted | 14 |

**OTHER MEATS**

| | |
|---|---|
| Venison | 3 |
| Beefalo | 5 |
| Rabbit | 6 |
| Tongue: beef, lamb, pork | 17 |

0   10   20   30   40   50
fat (grams)

\* Counts are based on 3-ounce servings.

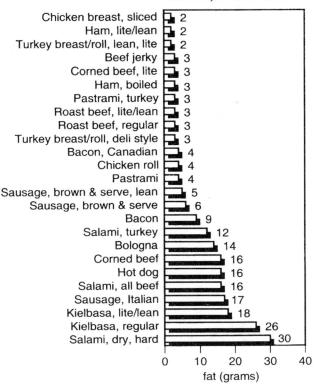

## Hi-Low Comparison Chart
(for Alphabetical Charts, see pages 1 - 82)

### MEATS, PROCESSED*

| Item | fat (grams) |
|---|---|
| Chicken breast, sliced | 2 |
| Ham, lite/lean | 2 |
| Turkey breast/roll, lean, lite | 2 |
| Beef jerky | 3 |
| Corned beef, lite | 3 |
| Ham, boiled | 3 |
| Pastrami, turkey | 3 |
| Roast beef, lite/lean | 3 |
| Roast beef, regular | 3 |
| Turkey breast/roll, deli style | 3 |
| Bacon, Canadian | 4 |
| Chicken roll | 4 |
| Pastrami | 4 |
| Sausage, brown & serve, lean | 5 |
| Sausage, brown & serve | 6 |
| Bacon | 9 |
| Salami, turkey | 12 |
| Bologna | 14 |
| Corned beef | 16 |
| Hot dog | 16 |
| Salami, all beef | 16 |
| Sausage, Italian | 17 |
| Kielbasa, lite/lean | 18 |
| Kielbasa, regular | 26 |
| Salami, dry, hard | 30 |

fat (grams)

* Counts are based on 3-ounce servings.

## Medications: COUGH DROPS & SYRUPS*

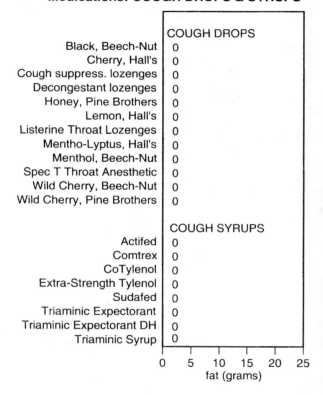

| | COUGH DROPS | |
|---|---|---|
| Black, Beech-Nut | 0 | |
| Cherry, Hall's | 0 | |
| Cough suppress. lozenges | 0 | |
| Decongestant lozenges | 0 | |
| Honey, Pine Brothers | 0 | |
| Lemon, Hall's | 0 | |
| Listerine Throat Lozenges | 0 | |
| Mentho-Lyptus, Hall's | 0 | |
| Menthol, Beech-Nut | 0 | |
| Spec T Throat Anesthetic | 0 | |
| Wild Cherry, Beech-Nut | 0 | |
| Wild Cherry, Pine Brothers | 0 | |
| | **COUGH SYRUPS** | |
| Actifed | 0 | |
| Comtrex | 0 | |
| CoTylenol | 0 | |
| Extra-Strength Tylenol | 0 | |
| Sudafed | 0 | |
| Triaminic Expectorant | 0 | |
| Triaminic Expectorant DH | 0 | |
| Triaminic Syrup | 0 | |

0   5   10   15   20   25
fat (grams)

\* Counts are based on one cough drop or on recommended
doses for adults.

## Medications: OVER-THE-COUNTER REMEDIES & VITAMINS AND MINERALS*

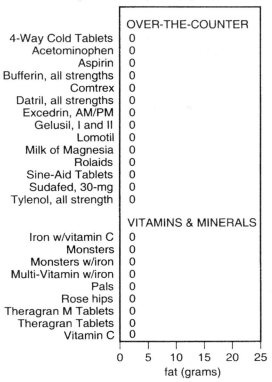

| | OVER-THE-COUNTER |
|---|---|
| 4-Way Cold Tablets | 0 |
| Acetominophen | 0 |
| Aspirin | 0 |
| Bufferin, all strengths | 0 |
| Comtrex | 0 |
| Datril, all strengths | 0 |
| Excedrin, AM/PM | 0 |
| Gelusil, I and II | 0 |
| Lomotil | 0 |
| Milk of Magnesia | 0 |
| Rolaids | 0 |
| Sine-Aid Tablets | 0 |
| Sudafed, 30-mg | 0 |
| Tylenol, all strength | 0 |
| | **VITAMINS & MINERALS** |
| Iron w/vitamin C | 0 |
| Monsters | 0 |
| Monsters w/iron | 0 |
| Multi-Vitamin w/iron | 0 |
| Pals | 0 |
| Rose hips | 0 |
| Theragran M Tablets | 0 |
| Theragran Tablets | 0 |
| Vitamin C | 0 |

0   5   10   15   20   25
fat (grams)

* Counts are based on recommended doses for adults.

129

## MISCELLANEOUS FOODS*

| Food | fat (grams) |
|------|------|
| Baking powder | 0 |
| Catsup | 0 |
| Chili powder | 0 |
| Cinnamon | 0 |
| Cocoa powder | 0 |
| Curry powder | 0 |
| Garlic powder | 0 |
| Gelatin, dry, 1 envelope | 0 |
| Ketchup | 0 |
| Mustard, w/ wine | 0 |
| Mustard, golden | 0 |
| Mustard, prepared yellow | 0 |
| Pepper, black | 0 |
| Pickles, dill, 1 medium | 0 |
| Pickles, fresh-pack, 2 slices | 0 |
| Pickles, sweet, 1 gherkin | 0 |
| Relish, sweet, chopped | 0 |
| Vinegar, balsamic | 0 |
| Vinegar, raspberry | 0 |
| Vinegar, red wine | 0 |
| Vinegar, white or cider | 0 |
| Yeast, 1 package | 0 |
| Olives, green, 3 medium | 2 |
| Olives, ripe, 3 medium | 2 |
| Chocolate, bitter baking | 8 |

fat (grams)

* Unless otherwise indicated, counts are based on
a one-tablespoon serving.

130

## NUTS, BEANS AND SEEDS*: Part 1

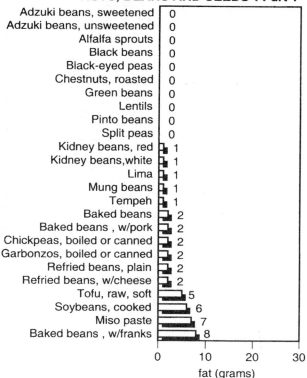

fat (grams)

* Unless otherwise indicated, counts are based on 1/2 cup
tofu or cooked beans or one-ounce servings of raw nuts or
seeds.

## NUTS, BEANS AND SEEDS\*: Part 2

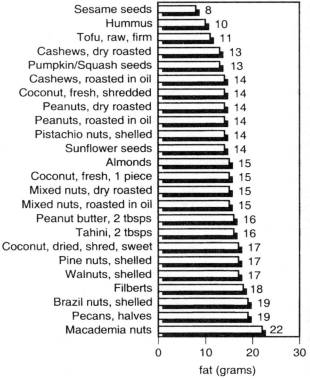

| | fat (grams) |
|---|---|
| Sesame seeds | 8 |
| Hummus | 10 |
| Tofu, raw, firm | 11 |
| Cashews, dry roasted | 13 |
| Pumpkin/Squash seeds | 13 |
| Cashews, roasted in oil | 14 |
| Coconut, fresh, shredded | 14 |
| Peanuts, dry roasted | 14 |
| Peanuts, roasted in oil | 14 |
| Pistachio nuts, shelled | 14 |
| Sunflower seeds | 14 |
| Almonds | 15 |
| Coconut, fresh, 1 piece | 15 |
| Mixed nuts, dry roasted | 15 |
| Mixed nuts, roasted in oil | 15 |
| Peanut butter, 2 tbsps | 16 |
| Tahini, 2 tbsps | 16 |
| Coconut, dried, shred, sweet | 17 |
| Pine nuts, shelled | 17 |
| Walnuts, shelled | 17 |
| Filberts | 18 |
| Brazil nuts, shelled | 19 |
| Pecans, halves | 19 |
| Macadamia nuts | 22 |

fat (grams)

\* Unless otherwise indicated, counts are based on 1/2 cup
tofu or cooked beans or one-ounce servings of raw nuts or
seeds.

## OILS AND FATS*

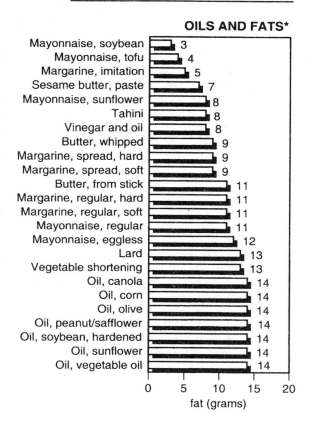

| | fat (grams) |
|---|---|
| Mayonnaise, soybean | 3 |
| Mayonnaise, tofu | 4 |
| Margarine, imitation | 5 |
| Sesame butter, paste | 7 |
| Mayonnaise, sunflower | 8 |
| Tahini | 8 |
| Vinegar and oil | 8 |
| Butter, whipped | 9 |
| Margarine, spread, hard | 9 |
| Margarine, spread, soft | 9 |
| Butter, from stick | 11 |
| Margarine, regular, hard | 11 |
| Margarine, regular, soft | 11 |
| Mayonnaise, regular | 11 |
| Mayonnaise, eggless | 12 |
| Lard | 13 |
| Vegetable shortening | 13 |
| Oil, canola | 14 |
| Oil, corn | 14 |
| Oil, olive | 14 |
| Oil, peanut/safflower | 14 |
| Oil, soybean, hardened | 14 |
| Oil, sunflower | 14 |
| Oil, vegetable oil | 14 |

* Counts are based on 1-tablespoon servings.

133

## PASTA, WHOLE GRAINS , RICE & NOODLES*, Part 1

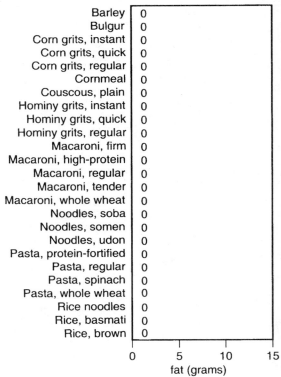

| | fat (grams) |
|---|---|
| Barley | 0 |
| Bulgur | 0 |
| Corn grits, instant | 0 |
| Corn grits, quick | 0 |
| Corn grits, regular | 0 |
| Cornmeal | 0 |
| Couscous, plain | 0 |
| Hominy grits, instant | 0 |
| Hominy grits, quick | 0 |
| Hominy grits, regular | 0 |
| Macaroni, firm | 0 |
| Macaroni, high-protein | 0 |
| Macaroni, regular | 0 |
| Macaroni, tender | 0 |
| Macaroni, whole wheat | 0 |
| Noodles, soba | 0 |
| Noodles, somen | 0 |
| Noodles, udon | 0 |
| Pasta, protein-fortified | 0 |
| Pasta, regular | 0 |
| Pasta, spinach | 0 |
| Pasta, whole wheat | 0 |
| Rice noodles | 0 |
| Rice, basmati | 0 |
| Rice, brown | 0 |

0　　　5　　　10　　　15
fat (grams)

\* Counts are based on cooked, 1/2-cup servings.

## PASTA, WHOLE GRAINS , RICE & NOODLES*, Part 2

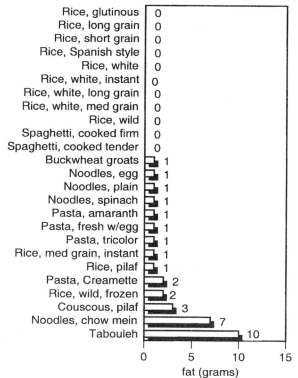

| | fat (grams) |
|---|---|
| Rice, glutinous | 0 |
| Rice, long grain | 0 |
| Rice, short grain | 0 |
| Rice, Spanish style | 0 |
| Rice, white | 0 |
| Rice, white, instant | 0 |
| Rice, white, long grain | 0 |
| Rice, white, med grain | 0 |
| Rice, wild | 0 |
| Spaghetti, cooked firm | 0 |
| Spaghetti, cooked tender | 0 |
| Buckwheat groats | 1 |
| Noodles, egg | 1 |
| Noodles, plain | 1 |
| Noodles, spinach | 1 |
| Pasta, amaranth | 1 |
| Pasta, fresh w/egg | 1 |
| Pasta, tricolor | 1 |
| Rice, med grain, instant | 1 |
| Rice, pilaf | 1 |
| Pasta, Creamette | 2 |
| Rice, wild, frozen | 2 |
| Couscous, pilaf | 3 |
| Noodles, chow mein | 7 |
| Tabouleh | 10 |

fat (grams)

* Counts are based on cooked, 1/2-cup servings.

135

## Poultry: CHICKEN, TURKEY, AND OTHER FOWL*

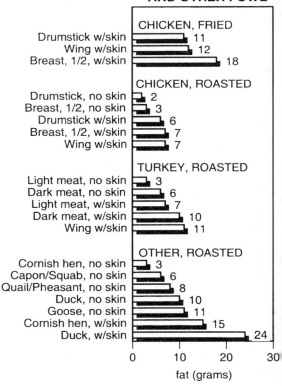

CHICKEN, FRIED
Drumstick w/skin — 11
Wing w/skin — 12
Breast, 1/2, w/skin — 18

CHICKEN, ROASTED
Drumstick, no skin — 2
Breast, 1/2, no skin — 3
Drumstick w/skin — 6
Breast, 1/2, w/skin — 7
Wing w/skin — 7

TURKEY, ROASTED
Light meat, no skin — 3
Dark meat, no skin — 6
Light meat, w/skin — 7
Dark meat, w/skin — 10
Wing w/skin — 11

OTHER, ROASTED
Cornish hen, no skin — 3
Capon/Squab, no skin — 6
Quail/Pheasant, no skin — 8
Duck, no skin — 10
Goose, no skin — 11
Cornish hen, w/skin — 15
Duck, w/skin — 24

0      10      20      30
fat (grams)

* Unless otherwise indicated, counts are based on 3-ounce
  servings.

## SALAD BAR CHOICES*

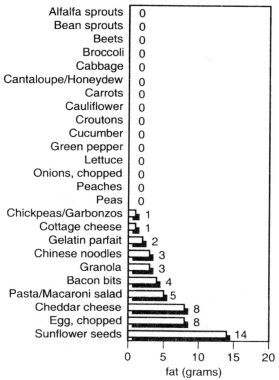

| Salad Bar Choice | fat (grams) |
|---|---|
| Alfalfa sprouts | 0 |
| Bean sprouts | 0 |
| Beets | 0 |
| Broccoli | 0 |
| Cabbage | 0 |
| Cantaloupe/Honeydew | 0 |
| Carrots | 0 |
| Cauliflower | 0 |
| Croutons | 0 |
| Cucumber | 0 |
| Green pepper | 0 |
| Lettuce | 0 |
| Onions, chopped | 0 |
| Peaches | 0 |
| Peas | 0 |
| Chickpeas/Garbonzos | 1 |
| Cottage cheese | 1 |
| Gelatin parfait | 2 |
| Chinese noodles | 3 |
| Granola | 3 |
| Bacon bits | 4 |
| Pasta/Macaroni salad | 5 |
| Cheddar cheese | 8 |
| Egg, chopped | 8 |
| Sunflower seeds | 14 |

fat (grams) — 0  5  10  15  20

\* Counts are based on one-quarter cup servings.

**SALAD DRESSING***

| Salad Dressing | fat (grams) |
|---|---|
| Italian, low-cal | 0 |
| Mayonnaise, lowfat dress. | 1 |
| Russian/Thous Island, low-cal | 1 |
| Blue cheese, low-cal | 2 |
| Creamy Italian, low-cal | 2 |
| French, low-cal | 2 |
| Honey mustard | 3 |
| Vinaigrette, low-cal | 3 |
| Miracle Whip, light | 4 |
| Oil & vinegar dressing | 4 |
| Garlic, regular | 5 |
| Mayonnaise, light | 5 |
| Russian/Thous Island, reg | 5 |
| Blue cheese, reg | 6 |
| Creamy Italian, regular | 6 |
| Vinaigrette, regular | 6 |
| Miracle Whip, regular | 7 |
| Onion & chives | 7 |
| Caesar | 8 |
| Garlic, creamy | 8 |
| Oil & vinegar | 8 |
| Ranch | 8 |
| French, regular | 9 |
| Italian, regular | 9 |
| Mayonnaise, reg | 11 |

fat (grams): 0 — 5 — 10 — 15

\* For ease of comparison, counts are based on single
tablespoon servings. Adjust counts to reflect quantities
consumed.

## SEAFOOD*, Part 1

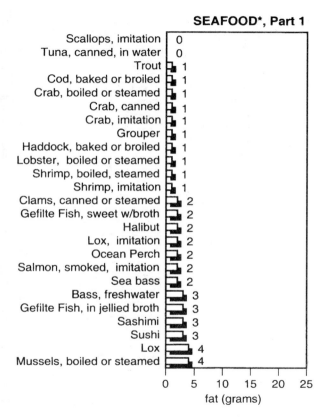

| Item | fat (grams) |
|------|-------------|
| Scallops, imitation | 0 |
| Tuna, canned, in water | 0 |
| Trout | 1 |
| Cod, baked or broiled | 1 |
| Crab, boiled or steamed | 1 |
| Crab, canned | 1 |
| Crab, imitation | 1 |
| Grouper | 1 |
| Haddock, baked or broiled | 1 |
| Lobster, boiled or steamed | 1 |
| Shrimp, boiled, steamed | 1 |
| Shrimp, imitation | 1 |
| Clams, canned or steamed | 2 |
| Gefilte Fish, sweet w/broth | 2 |
| Halibut | 2 |
| Lox, imitation | 2 |
| Ocean Perch | 2 |
| Salmon, smoked, imitation | 2 |
| Sea bass | 2 |
| Bass, freshwater | 3 |
| Gefilte Fish, in jellied broth | 3 |
| Sashimi | 3 |
| Sushi | 3 |
| Lox | 4 |
| Mussels, boiled or steamed | 4 |

fat (grams) — 0 5 10 15 20 25

* Counts are based on 3-ounce servings. Canned seafood
items are assumed to be drained.

## SEAFOOD*, Part 2

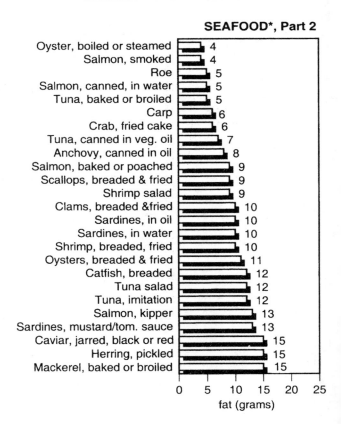

| | fat (grams) |
|---|---|
| Oyster, boiled or steamed | 4 |
| Salmon, smoked | 4 |
| Roe | 5 |
| Salmon, canned, in water | 5 |
| Tuna, baked or broiled | 5 |
| Carp | 6 |
| Crab, fried cake | 6 |
| Tuna, canned in veg. oil | 7 |
| Anchovy, canned in oil | 8 |
| Salmon, baked or poached | 9 |
| Scallops, breaded & fried | 9 |
| Shrimp salad | 9 |
| Clams, breaded &fried | 10 |
| Sardines, in oil | 10 |
| Sardines, in water | 10 |
| Shrimp, breaded, fried | 10 |
| Oysters, breaded & fried | 11 |
| Catfish, breaded | 12 |
| Tuna salad | 12 |
| Tuna, imitation | 12 |
| Salmon, kipper | 13 |
| Sardines, mustard/tom. sauce | 13 |
| Caviar, jarred, black or red | 15 |
| Herring, pickled | 15 |
| Mackerel, baked or broiled | 15 |

0   5   10   15   20   25
fat (grams)

\* Counts are based on 3-ounce servings. Canned seafood
items are assumed to be drained.

## SNACKS: AND CHIPS: Part 1*

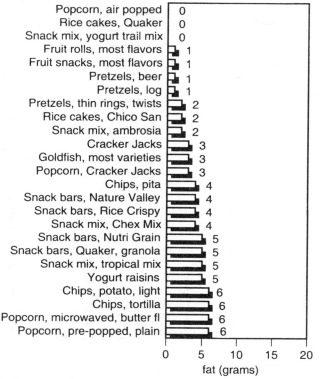

| Snack | fat (grams) |
|---|---|
| Popcorn, air popped | 0 |
| Rice cakes, Quaker | 0 |
| Snack mix, yogurt trail mix | 0 |
| Fruit rolls, most flavors | 1 |
| Fruit snacks, most flavors | 1 |
| Pretzels, beer | 1 |
| Pretzels, log | 1 |
| Pretzels, thin rings, twists | 2 |
| Rice cakes, Chico San | 2 |
| Snack mix, ambrosia | 2 |
| Cracker Jacks | 3 |
| Goldfish, most varieties | 3 |
| Popcorn, Cracker Jacks | 3 |
| Chips, pita | 4 |
| Snack bars, Nature Valley | 4 |
| Snack bars, Rice Crispy | 4 |
| Snack mix, Chex Mix | 4 |
| Snack bars, Nutri Grain | 5 |
| Snack bars, Quaker, granola | 5 |
| Snack mix, tropical mix | 5 |
| Yogurt raisins | 5 |
| Chips, potato, light | 6 |
| Chips, tortilla | 6 |
| Popcorn, microwaved, butter fl | 6 |
| Popcorn, pre-popped, plain | 6 |

fat (grams)

\* For ease of comparison, counts are based on one-ounce
servings. For popcorn, 1 ounce unpopped = 2 cups popped.
Adjust count to reflect amount consumed.

## SNACKS AND CHIPS: Part 2*

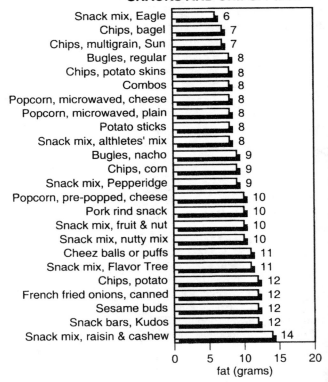

| | fat (grams) |
|---|---|
| Snack mix, Eagle | 6 |
| Chips, bagel | 7 |
| Chips, multigrain, Sun | 7 |
| Bugles, regular | 8 |
| Chips, potato skins | 8 |
| Combos | 8 |
| Popcorn, microwaved, cheese | 8 |
| Popcorn, microwaved, plain | 8 |
| Potato sticks | 8 |
| Snack mix, althletes' mix | 8 |
| Bugles, nacho | 9 |
| Chips, corn | 9 |
| Snack mix, Pepperidge | 9 |
| Popcorn, pre-popped, cheese | 10 |
| Pork rind snack | 10 |
| Snack mix, fruit & nut | 10 |
| Snack mix, nutty mix | 10 |
| Cheez balls or puffs | 11 |
| Snack mix, Flavor Tree | 11 |
| Chips, potato | 12 |
| French fried onions, canned | 12 |
| Sesame buds | 12 |
| Snack bars, Kudos | 12 |
| Snack mix, raisin & cashew | 14 |

*   For ease of comparison, counts are based on one-ounce
    servings. For popcorn, 1 ounce unpopped = 2 cups popped.
    Adjust count to reflect amount consumed.

## SOUP*: Part 1

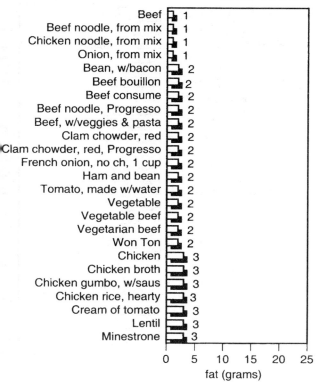

| Soup | fat (grams) |
|------|-------------|
| Beef | 1 |
| Beef noodle, from mix | 1 |
| Chicken noodle, from mix | 1 |
| Onion, from mix | 1 |
| Bean, w/bacon | 2 |
| Beef bouillon | 2 |
| Beef consume | 2 |
| Beef noodle, Progresso | 2 |
| Beef, w/veggies & pasta | 2 |
| Clam chowder, red | 2 |
| Clam chowder, red, Progresso | 2 |
| French onion, no ch, 1 cup | 2 |
| Ham and bean | 2 |
| Tomato, made w/water | 2 |
| Vegetable | 2 |
| Vegetable beef | 2 |
| Vegetarian beef | 2 |
| Won Ton | 2 |
| Chicken | 3 |
| Chicken broth | 3 |
| Chicken gumbo, w/saus | 3 |
| Chicken rice, hearty | 3 |
| Cream of tomato | 3 |
| Lentil | 3 |
| Minestrone | 3 |

fat (grams) — scale: 0 5 10 15 20 25

* Unless otherwise indicated, counts are based on one-cup servings.

143

**SOUP\*: Part 2**

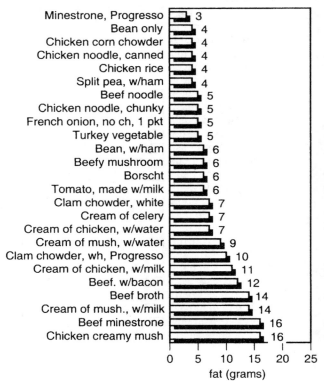

| Soup | fat (grams) |
|------|-------------|
| Minestrone, Progresso | 3 |
| Bean only | 4 |
| Chicken corn chowder | 4 |
| Chicken noodle, canned | 4 |
| Chicken rice | 4 |
| Split pea, w/ham | 4 |
| Beef noodle | 5 |
| Chicken noodle, chunky | 5 |
| French onion, no ch, 1 pkt | 5 |
| Turkey vegetable | 5 |
| Bean, w/ham | 6 |
| Beefy mushroom | 6 |
| Borscht | 6 |
| Tomato, made w/milk | 6 |
| Clam chowder, white | 7 |
| Cream of celery | 7 |
| Cream of chicken, w/water | 7 |
| Cream of mush, w/water | 9 |
| Clam chowder, wh, Progresso | 10 |
| Cream of chicken, w/milk | 11 |
| Beef. w/bacon | 12 |
| Beef broth | 14 |
| Cream of mush., w/milk | 14 |
| Beef minestrone | 16 |
| Chicken creamy mush | 16 |

fat (grams) — 0 5 10 15 20 25

\* Unless otherwise indicated, counts are based on one-cup servings.

## Sweets: CAKES*, Part 1

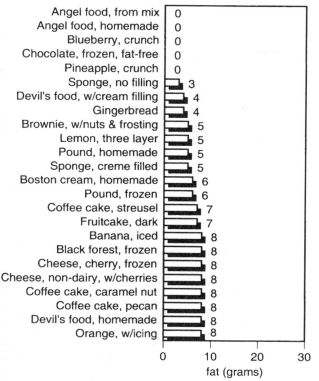

| | fat (grams) |
|---|---|
| Angel food, from mix | 0 |
| Angel food, homemade | 0 |
| Blueberry, crunch | 0 |
| Chocolate, frozen, fat-free | 0 |
| Pineapple, crunch | 0 |
| Sponge, no filling | 3 |
| Devil's food, w/cream filling | 4 |
| Gingerbread | 4 |
| Brownie, w/nuts & frosting | 5 |
| Lemon, three layer | 5 |
| Pound, homemade | 5 |
| Sponge, creme filled | 5 |
| Boston cream, homemade | 6 |
| Pound, frozen | 6 |
| Coffee cake, streusel | 7 |
| Fruitcake, dark | 7 |
| Banana, iced | 8 |
| Black forest, frozen | 8 |
| Cheese, cherry, frozen | 8 |
| Cheese, non-dairy, w/cherries | 8 |
| Coffee cake, caramel nut | 8 |
| Coffee cake, pecan | 8 |
| Devil's food, homemade | 8 |
| Orange, w/icing | 8 |

* Counts are based on average-size pieces and slices,
  where appropriate, as indicated on package.

145

## Sweets: CAKES*, Part 2

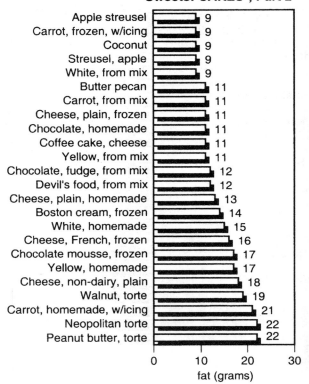

| Cake | fat (grams) |
|---|---|
| Apple streusel | 9 |
| Carrot, frozen, w/icing | 9 |
| Coconut | 9 |
| Streusel, apple | 9 |
| White, from mix | 9 |
| Butter pecan | 11 |
| Carrot, from mix | 11 |
| Cheese, plain, frozen | 11 |
| Chocolate, homemade | 11 |
| Coffee cake, cheese | 11 |
| Yellow, from mix | 11 |
| Chocolate, fudge, from mix | 12 |
| Devil's food, from mix | 12 |
| Cheese, plain, homemade | 13 |
| Boston cream, frozen | 14 |
| White, homemade | 15 |
| Cheese, French, frozen | 16 |
| Chocolate mousse, frozen | 17 |
| Yellow, homemade | 17 |
| Cheese, non-dairy, plain | 18 |
| Walnut, torte | 19 |
| Carrot, homemade, w/icing | 21 |
| Neopolitan torte | 22 |
| Peanut butter, torte | 22 |

fat (grams)

\* Counts are based on average-size servings.

## Sweets: SNACK CAKES*

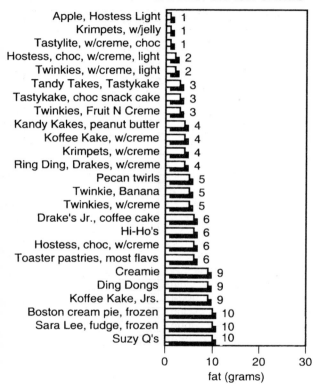

| Snack Cake | fat (grams) |
|---|---|
| Apple, Hostess Light | 1 |
| Krimpets, w/jelly | 1 |
| Tastylite, w/creme, choc | 1 |
| Hostess, choc, w/creme, light | 2 |
| Twinkies, w/creme, light | 2 |
| Tandy Takes, Tastykake | 3 |
| Tastykake, choc snack cake | 3 |
| Twinkies, Fruit N Creme | 3 |
| Kandy Kakes, peanut butter | 4 |
| Koffee Kake, w/creme | 4 |
| Krimpets, w/creme | 4 |
| Ring Ding, Drakes, w/creme | 4 |
| Pecan twirls | 5 |
| Twinkie, Banana | 5 |
| Twinkies, w/creme | 5 |
| Drake's Jr., coffee cake | 6 |
| Hi-Ho's | 6 |
| Hostess, choc, w/creme | 6 |
| Toaster pastries, most flavs | 6 |
| Creamie | 9 |
| Ding Dongs | 9 |
| Koffee Kake, Jrs. | 9 |
| Boston cream pie, frozen | 10 |
| Sara Lee, fudge, frozen | 10 |
| Suzy Q's | 10 |

fat (grams)

* Counts are based on average-size pieces and slices,
  where appropriate, as indicated on package.

147

## Sweets: CANDY*: Part 1

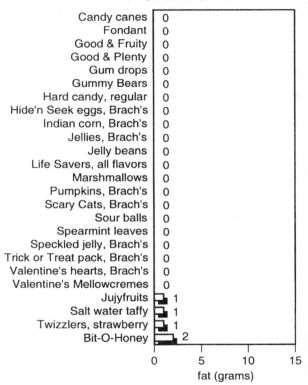

| | fat (grams) |
|---|---|
| Candy canes | 0 |
| Fondant | 0 |
| Good & Fruity | 0 |
| Good & Plenty | 0 |
| Gum drops | 0 |
| Gummy Bears | 0 |
| Hard candy, regular | 0 |
| Hide'n Seek eggs, Brach's | 0 |
| Indian corn, Brach's | 0 |
| Jellies, Brach's | 0 |
| Jelly beans | 0 |
| Life Savers, all flavors | 0 |
| Marshmallows | 0 |
| Pumpkins, Brach's | 0 |
| Scary Cats, Brach's | 0 |
| Sour balls | 0 |
| Spearmint leaves | 0 |
| Speckled jelly, Brach's | 0 |
| Trick or Treat pack, Brach's | 0 |
| Valentine's hearts, Brach's | 0 |
| Valentine's Mellowcremes | 0 |
| Jujyfruits | 1 |
| Salt water taffy | 1 |
| Twizzlers, strawberry | 1 |
| Bit-O-Honey | 2 |

\* For ease of comparison, counts are based on one-ounce
servings. Adjust counts to reflect quantities consumed.

## Sweets: CANDY*, Part 2

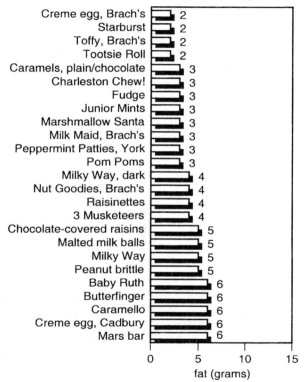

| Candy | fat (grams) |
|---|---|
| Creme egg, Brach's | 2 |
| Starburst | 2 |
| Toffy, Brach's | 2 |
| Tootsie Roll | 2 |
| Caramels, plain/chocolate | 3 |
| Charleston Chew! | 3 |
| Fudge | 3 |
| Junior Mints | 3 |
| Marshmallow Santa | 3 |
| Milk Maid, Brach's | 3 |
| Peppermint Patties, York | 3 |
| Pom Poms | 3 |
| Milky Way, dark | 4 |
| Nut Goodies, Brach's | 4 |
| Raisinettes | 4 |
| 3 Musketeers | 4 |
| Chocolate-covered raisins | 5 |
| Malted milk balls | 5 |
| Milky Way | 5 |
| Peanut brittle | 5 |
| Baby Ruth | 6 |
| Butterfinger | 6 |
| Caramello | 6 |
| Creme egg, Cadbury | 6 |
| Mars bar | 6 |

fat (grams)

\* For ease of comparison, counts are based on one-ounce
servings. Adjust counts to reflect quantities consumed.

## Sweets: CANDY*, Part 3

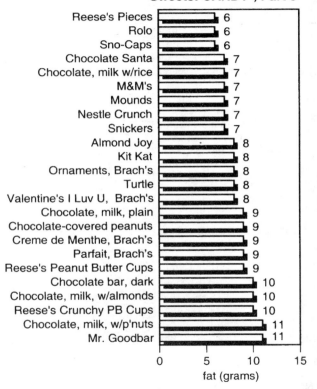

| | fat (grams) |
|---|---|
| Reese's Pieces | 6 |
| Rolo | 6 |
| Sno-Caps | 6 |
| Chocolate Santa | 7 |
| Chocolate, milk w/rice | 7 |
| M&M's | 7 |
| Mounds | 7 |
| Nestle Crunch | 7 |
| Snickers | 7 |
| Almond Joy | 8 |
| Kit Kat | 8 |
| Ornaments, Brach's | 8 |
| Turtle | 8 |
| Valentine's I Luv U, Brach's | 8 |
| Chocolate, milk, plain | 9 |
| Chocolate-covered peanuts | 9 |
| Creme de Menthe, Brach's | 9 |
| Parfait, Brach's | 9 |
| Reese's Peanut Butter Cups | 9 |
| Chocolate bar, dark | 10 |
| Chocolate, milk, w/almonds | 10 |
| Reese's Crunchy PB Cups | 10 |
| Chocolate, milk, w/p'nuts | 11 |
| Mr. Goodbar | 11 |

* For ease of comparison, counts are based on one-ounce
servings. Adjust counts to reflect quantities consumed.

## Sweets: COOKIES*, Part 1

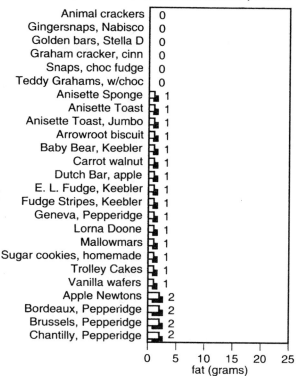

| | fat (grams) |
|---|---|
| Animal crackers | 0 |
| Gingersnaps, Nabisco | 0 |
| Golden bars, Stella D | 0 |
| Graham cracker, cinn | 0 |
| Snaps, choc fudge | 0 |
| Teddy Grahams, w/choc | 0 |
| Anisette Sponge | 1 |
| Anisette Toast | 1 |
| Anisette Toast, Jumbo | 1 |
| Arrowroot biscuit | 1 |
| Baby Bear, Keebler | 1 |
| Carrot walnut | 1 |
| Dutch Bar, apple | 1 |
| E. L. Fudge, Keebler | 1 |
| Fudge Stripes, Keebler | 1 |
| Geneva, Pepperidge | 1 |
| Lorna Doone | 1 |
| Mallowmars | 1 |
| Sugar cookies, homemade | 1 |
| Trolley Cakes | 1 |
| Vanilla wafers | 1 |
| Apple Newtons | 2 |
| Bordeaux, Pepperidge | 2 |
| Brussels, Pepperidge | 2 |
| Chantilly, Pepperidge | 2 |

fat (grams): 0  5  10  15  20  25

* NOTE: For ease of comparison, counts are based on
single cookie servings. When more than one cookie is
consumed, counts should be adjusted accordingly.

## Sweets: COOKIES*, Part 2

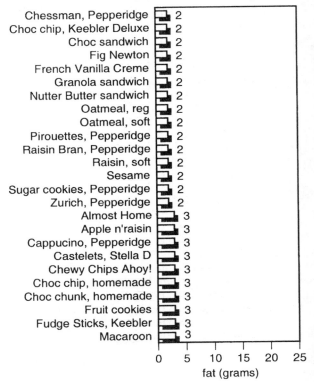

| | fat (grams) |
|---|---|
| Chessman, Pepperidge | 2 |
| Choc chip, Keebler Deluxe | 2 |
| Choc sandwich | 2 |
| Fig Newton | 2 |
| French Vanilla Creme | 2 |
| Granola sandwich | 2 |
| Nutter Butter sandwich | 2 |
| Oatmeal, reg | 2 |
| Oatmeal, soft | 2 |
| Pirouettes, Pepperidge | 2 |
| Raisin Bran, Pepperidge | 2 |
| Raisin, soft | 2 |
| Sesame | 2 |
| Sugar cookies, Pepperidge | 2 |
| Zurich, Pepperidge | 2 |
| Almost Home | 3 |
| Apple n'raisin | 3 |
| Cappucino, Pepperidge | 3 |
| Castelets, Stella D | 3 |
| Chewy Chips Ahoy! | 3 |
| Choc chip, homemade | 3 |
| Choc chunk, homemade | 3 |
| Fruit cookies | 3 |
| Fudge Sticks, Keebler | 3 |
| Macaroon | 3 |

0   5   10   15   20   25
fat (grams)

\* NOTE: For ease of comparison, counts are based on
single cookie servings. When more than one cookie is
consumed, counts should be adjusted accordingly.

## Sweets: COOKIES, Part 3

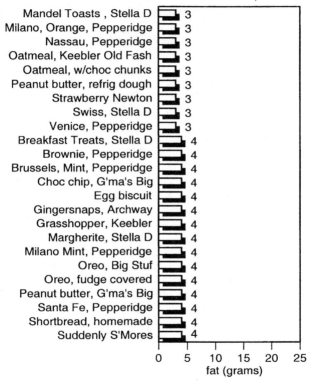

| | fat (grams) |
|---|---|
| Mandel Toasts , Stella D | 3 |
| Milano, Orange, Pepperidge | 3 |
| Nassau, Pepperidge | 3 |
| Oatmeal, Keebler Old Fash | 3 |
| Oatmeal, w/choc chunks | 3 |
| Peanut butter, refrig dough | 3 |
| Strawberry Newton | 3 |
| Swiss, Stella D | 3 |
| Venice, Pepperidge | 3 |
| Breakfast Treats, Stella D | 4 |
| Brownie, Pepperidge | 4 |
| Brussels, Mint, Pepperidge | 4 |
| Choc chip, G'ma's Big | 4 |
| Egg biscuit | 4 |
| Gingersnaps, Archway | 4 |
| Grasshopper, Keebler | 4 |
| Margherite, Stella D | 4 |
| Milano Mint, Pepperidge | 4 |
| Oreo, Big Stuf | 4 |
| Oreo, fudge covered | 4 |
| Peanut butter, G'ma's Big | 4 |
| Santa Fe, Pepperidge | 4 |
| Shortbread, homemade | 4 |
| Suddenly S'Mores | 4 |

0    5    10    15    20    25
fat (grams)

\* NOTE: For ease of comparison, counts are based on
single cookie servings. When more than one cookie is
consumed, counts should be adjusted accordingly.

## Sweets: COOKIES*, Part 4

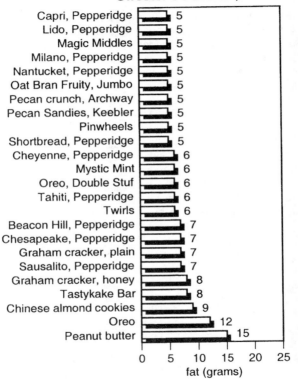

| Cookie | fat (grams) |
|---|---|
| Capri, Pepperidge | 5 |
| Lido, Pepperidge | 5 |
| Magic Middles | 5 |
| Milano, Pepperidge | 5 |
| Nantucket, Pepperidge | 5 |
| Oat Bran Fruity, Jumbo | 5 |
| Pecan crunch, Archway | 5 |
| Pecan Sandies, Keebler | 5 |
| Pinwheels | 5 |
| Shortbread, Pepperidge | 5 |
| Cheyenne, Pepperidge | 6 |
| Mystic Mint | 6 |
| Oreo, Double Stuf | 6 |
| Tahiti, Pepperidge | 6 |
| Twirls | 6 |
| Beacon Hill, Pepperidge | 7 |
| Chesapeake, Pepperidge | 7 |
| Graham cracker, plain | 7 |
| Sausalito, Pepperidge | 7 |
| Graham cracker, honey | 8 |
| Tastykake Bar | 8 |
| Chinese almond cookies | 9 |
| Oreo | 12 |
| Peanut butter | 15 |

fat (grams)

* NOTE: For ease of comparison, counts are based on
single cookie servings. When more than one cookie is
consumed, counts should be adjusted accordingly.

Hi-Low Comparison Chart
(for Alphabetical Charts, see pages 1 - 82)

**Sweets: DONUTS\***

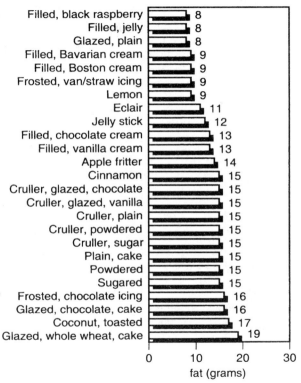

| Donut | fat (grams) |
|---|---|
| Filled, black raspberry | 8 |
| Filled, jelly | 8 |
| Glazed, plain | 8 |
| Filled, Bavarian cream | 9 |
| Filled, Boston cream | 9 |
| Frosted, van/straw icing | 9 |
| Lemon | 9 |
| Eclair | 11 |
| Jelly stick | 12 |
| Filled, chocolate cream | 13 |
| Filled, vanilla cream | 13 |
| Apple fritter | 14 |
| Cinnamon | 15 |
| Cruller, glazed, chocolate | 15 |
| Cruller, glazed, vanilla | 15 |
| Cruller, plain | 15 |
| Cruller, powdered | 15 |
| Cruller, sugar | 15 |
| Plain, cake | 15 |
| Powdered | 15 |
| Sugared | 15 |
| Frosted, chocolate icing | 16 |
| Glazed, chocolate, cake | 16 |
| Coconut, toasted | 17 |
| Glazed, whole wheat, cake | 19 |

fat (grams)

\* Counts are based on average-size donuts.

155

## Sweets: GUM & MINTS*

| | fat (grams) |
|---|---|
| **GUM** | |
| Beech-Nut | 0 |
| Beechies | 0 |
| Big Red | 0 |
| Bubble Care Free | 0 |
| Bubble Yum | 0 |
| Bubblicious | 0 |
| Care Free | 0 |
| Chewels | 0 |
| Chiclets | 0 |
| Dentyne | 0 |
| Dentyne, sugarless | 0 |
| Doublemint | 0 |
| Freedent | 0 |
| Freshen-Up | 0 |
| Hubba Bubba | 0 |
| Juicy Fruit | 0 |
| Wrigley's Spearmint | 0 |
| **MINTS** | |
| Breathsavers, spearmint | 0 |
| Chlorets | 0 |
| Tic Tac | 0 |

0   1   2   3   4   5
fat (grams)

* Counts are based on single sticks and mints.

**Sweets: ICE CREAM\***

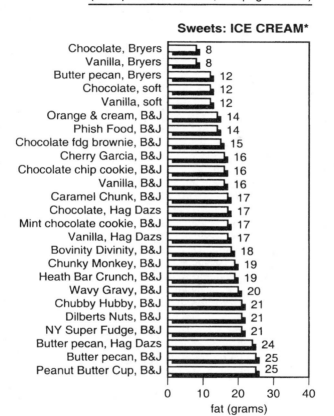

| Item | fat (grams) |
|------|-------------|
| Chocolate, Bryers | 8 |
| Vanilla, Bryers | 8 |
| Butter pecan, Bryers | 12 |
| Chocolate, soft | 12 |
| Vanilla, soft | 12 |
| Orange & cream, B&J | 14 |
| Phish Food, B&J | 14 |
| Chocolate fdg brownie, B&J | 15 |
| Cherry Garcia, B&J | 16 |
| Chocolate chip cookie, B&J | 16 |
| Vanilla, B&J | 16 |
| Caramel Chunk, B&J | 17 |
| Chocolate, Hag Dazs | 17 |
| Mint chocolate cookie, B&J | 17 |
| Vanilla, Hag Dazs | 17 |
| Bovinity Divinity, B&J | 18 |
| Chunky Monkey, B&J | 19 |
| Heath Bar Crunch, B&J | 19 |
| Wavy Gravy, B&J | 20 |
| Chubby Hubby, B&J | 21 |
| Dilberts Nuts, B&J | 21 |
| NY Super Fudge, B&J | 21 |
| Butter pecan, Hag Dazs | 24 |
| Butter pecan, B&J | 25 |
| Peanut Butter Cup, B&J | 25 |

fat (grams)

\* Counts are based on one-half cup servings. "B&J"
designates Ben & Jerry's brand.

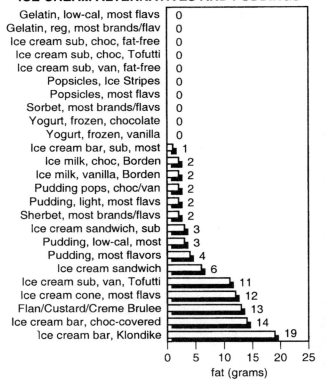

## Sweets: ICE CREAM CONES & BARS,
## ICE CREAM ALTERNATIVES AND PUDDINGS*

| | fat (grams) |
|---|---|
| Gelatin, low-cal, most flavs | 0 |
| Gelatin, reg, most brands/flav | 0 |
| Ice cream sub, choc, fat-free | 0 |
| Ice cream sub, choc, Tofutti | 0 |
| Ice cream sub, van, fat-free | 0 |
| Popsicles, Ice Stripes | 0 |
| Popsicles, most flavs | 0 |
| Sorbet, most brands/flavs | 0 |
| Yogurt, frozen, chocolate | 0 |
| Yogurt, frozen, vanilla | 0 |
| Ice cream bar, sub, most | 1 |
| Ice milk, choc, Borden | 2 |
| Ice milk, vanilla, Borden | 2 |
| Pudding pops, choc/van | 2 |
| Pudding, light, most flavs | 2 |
| Sherbet, most brands/flavs | 2 |
| Ice cream sandwich, sub | 3 |
| Pudding, low-cal, most | 3 |
| Pudding, most flavors | 4 |
| Ice cream sandwich | 6 |
| Ice cream sub, van, Tofutti | 11 |
| Ice cream cone, most flavs | 12 |
| Flan/Custard/Creme Brulee | 13 |
| Ice cream bar, choc-covered | 14 |
| Ice cream bar, Klondike | 19 |

* Counts are based on average- or one-half cup servings.
"Sub" designates non-dairy, ice cream substitute.

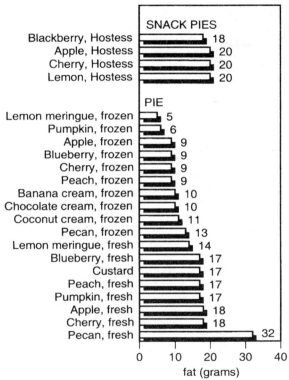

Hi-Low Comparison Chart
(for Alphabetical Charts, see pages 1 - 82)

**Sweets: PIES\***

SNACK PIES

| | |
|---|---|
| Blackberry, Hostess | 18 |
| Apple, Hostess | 20 |
| Cherry, Hostess | 20 |
| Lemon, Hostess | 20 |

PIE

| | |
|---|---|
| Lemon meringue, frozen | 5 |
| Pumpkin, frozen | 6 |
| Apple, frozen | 9 |
| Blueberry, frozen | 9 |
| Cherry, frozen | 9 |
| Peach, frozen | 9 |
| Banana cream, frozen | 10 |
| Chocolate cream, frozen | 10 |
| Coconut cream, frozen | 11 |
| Pecan, frozen | 13 |
| Lemon meringue, fresh | 14 |
| Blueberry, fresh | 17 |
| Custard | 17 |
| Peach, fresh | 17 |
| Pumpkin, fresh | 17 |
| Apple, fresh | 18 |
| Cherry, fresh | 18 |
| Pecan, fresh | 32 |

0   10   20   30   40
fat (grams)

\* Counts are based on average-size pieces and slices,
where appropriate, as indicated on package.

159

## Sweets: SUGARS, SYRUPS, TOPPINGS AND JAMS*

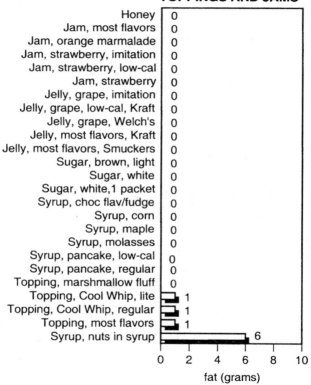

| | fat (grams) |
|---|---|
| Honey | 0 |
| Jam, most flavors | 0 |
| Jam, orange marmalade | 0 |
| Jam, strawberry, imitation | 0 |
| Jam, strawberry, low-cal | 0 |
| Jam, strawberry | 0 |
| Jelly, grape, imitation | 0 |
| Jelly, grape, low-cal, Kraft | 0 |
| Jelly, grape, Welch's | 0 |
| Jelly, most flavors, Kraft | 0 |
| Jelly, most flavors, Smuckers | 0 |
| Sugar, brown, light | 0 |
| Sugar, white | 0 |
| Sugar, white, 1 packet | 0 |
| Syrup, choc flav/fudge | 0 |
| Syrup, corn | 0 |
| Syrup, maple | 0 |
| Syrup, molasses | 0 |
| Syrup, pancake, low-cal | 0 |
| Syrup, pancake, regular | 0 |
| Topping, marshmallow fluff | 0 |
| Topping, Cool Whip, lite | 1 |
| Topping, Cool Whip, regular | 1 |
| Topping, most flavors | 1 |
| Syrup, nuts in syrup | 6 |

0   2   4   6   8   10
fat (grams)

\* Counts are based on single-tablespoon servings. Jams and preserves can be assumed to have equal values.

Hi-Low Comparison Chart
(for Alphabetical Charts, see pages 1 - 82)

## VEGETABLES*, Part 1

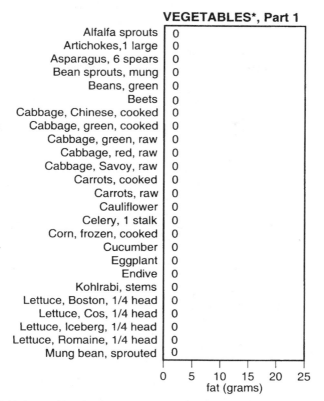

| | fat (grams) |
|---|---|
| Alfalfa sprouts | 0 |
| Artichokes, 1 large | 0 |
| Asparagus, 6 spears | 0 |
| Bean sprouts, mung | 0 |
| Beans, green | 0 |
| Beets | 0 |
| Cabbage, Chinese, cooked | 0 |
| Cabbage, green, cooked | 0 |
| Cabbage, green, raw | 0 |
| Cabbage, red, raw | 0 |
| Cabbage, Savoy, raw | 0 |
| Carrots, cooked | 0 |
| Carrots, raw | 0 |
| Cauliflower | 0 |
| Celery, 1 stalk | 0 |
| Corn, frozen, cooked | 0 |
| Cucumber | 0 |
| Eggplant | 0 |
| Endive | 0 |
| Kohlrabi, stems | 0 |
| Lettuce, Boston, 1/4 head | 0 |
| Lettuce, Cos, 1/4 head | 0 |
| Lettuce, Iceberg, 1/4 head | 0 |
| Lettuce, Romaine, 1/4 head | 0 |
| Mung bean, sprouted | 0 |

0   5   10   15   20   25
fat (grams)

\* Unless otherwise indicated, counts are based on one-cup servings. For vegetable juices, see the Fruits & Juices section.

## VEGETABLES*, Part 2

| | fat (grams) |
|---|---|
| Mushrooms, raw | 0 |
| Okra pods, 3 pods | 0 |
| Onions , cooked | 0 |
| Onions , raw | 0 |
| Parsnips | 0 |
| Pea pods, Chinese, cooked | 0 |
| Peppers, green, raw | 0 |
| Peppers, hot chili, 6 | 0 |
| Peppers, red, raw | 0 |
| Plantain, cooked & sliced | 0 |
| Potato, baked, 1 medium | 0 |
| Potato, sweet | 0 |
| Radishes, raw, 5 large | 0 |
| Sauerkraut | 0 |
| Seaweed, kelp, raw | 0 |
| Spinach, cooked | 0 |
| Spinach, raw | 0 |
| Tomato puree | 0 |
| Tomato sauce | 0 |
| Turnip greens | 0 |
| Turnips, cooked | 0 |
| Water chestnuts, canned | 0 |
| Bamboo shoots | 1 |
| Broccoli, 1 spear | 1 |
| Brussels sprouts | 1 |

0    5    10    15    20    25
fat (grams)

* Unless otherwise indicated, counts are based on one-cup
servings. For vegetable juices, see the Fruits & Juices
section.

162

## VEGETABLES*, Part 3

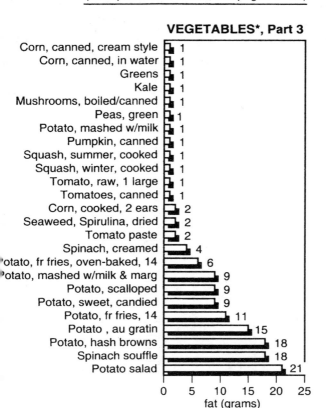

| | fat (grams) |
|---|---|
| Corn, canned, cream style | 1 |
| Corn, canned, in water | 1 |
| Greens | 1 |
| Kale | 1 |
| Mushrooms, boiled/canned | 1 |
| Peas, green | 1 |
| Potato, mashed w/milk | 1 |
| Pumpkin, canned | 1 |
| Squash, summer, cooked | 1 |
| Squash, winter, cooked | 1 |
| Tomato, raw, 1 large | 1 |
| Tomatoes, canned | 1 |
| Corn, cooked, 2 ears | 2 |
| Seaweed, Spirulina, dried | 2 |
| Tomato paste | 2 |
| Spinach, creamed | 4 |
| Potato, fr fries, oven-baked, 14 | 6 |
| Potato, mashed w/milk & marg | 9 |
| Potato, scalloped | 9 |
| Potato, sweet, candied | 9 |
| Potato, fr fries, 14 | 11 |
| Potato , au gratin | 15 |
| Potato, hash browns | 18 |
| Spinach souffle | 18 |
| Potato salad | 21 |

*   Unless otherwise indicated, counts are based on one-cup
    servings. For vegetable juices, see the Fruits & Juices
    section.

## VEGETARIAN CHOICES*

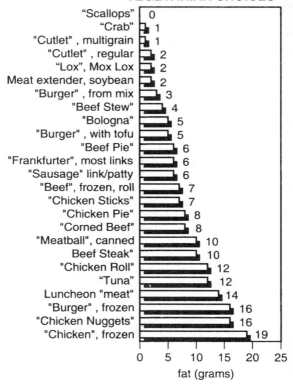

| | fat (grams) |
|---|---|
| "Scallops" | 0 |
| "Crab" | 1 |
| "Cutlet", multigrain | 1 |
| "Cutlet", regular | 2 |
| "Lox", Mox Lox | 2 |
| Meat extender, soybean | 2 |
| "Burger", from mix | 3 |
| "Beef Stew" | 4 |
| "Bologna" | 5 |
| "Burger", with tofu | 5 |
| "Beef Pie" | 6 |
| "Frankfurter", most links | 6 |
| "Sausage" link/patty | 6 |
| "Beef", frozen, roll | 7 |
| "Chicken Sticks" | 7 |
| "Chicken Pie" | 8 |
| "Corned Beef" | 8 |
| "Meatball", canned | 10 |
| Beef Steak" | 10 |
| "Chicken Roll" | 12 |
| "Tuna" | 12 |
| Luncheon "meat" | 14 |
| "Burger", frozen | 16 |
| "Chicken Nuggets" | 16 |
| "Chicken", frozen | 19 |

\* Made from tofu, textured vegetable protein or a combination of both. Counts are based on 3-ounce servings.